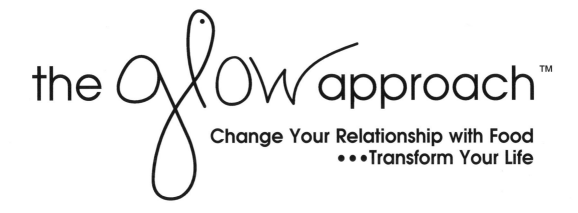

the glow approach™

Change Your Relationship with Food
•••Transform Your Life

Lyn Shroyer, EdD

glow and company publishing

Cover design and book layout by Shari Gannon and
edited by Toby Kane of Krave Branding, LLC.

Book photo credits.
Alexskopje. Shutterstock. Photo ID: 341665112. Retrieved from http://www.shutterstock.com.
Calkins, B. Shutterstock. Photo ID: 85277137. Retrieved from http://www.shutterstock.com.
DeeaF. Shutterstock. Photo ID: 407675521. Retrieved from http://www.shutterstock.com.
Frazao, G. Shutterstock. Photo ID: 344266346. Retrieved from http://www.shutterstock.com.
Glisic, A. Shutterstock. Photo ID: 358925636. Retrieved from http://www.shutterstock.com.
Maerz, M. Shutterstock. Photo ID: 264221285. Retrieved from http://www.shutterstock.com.
Udra11. Shutterstock. Photo ID: 335916848. Retrieved from http://www.shutterstock.com.

Disclaimer

The information contained in this book is for educational and informational purposes only, and is available to you as a self-help tool. It is not intended to be a substitute for professional advice, diagnosis, or treatment that can be provided by your physician, therapist, dietitian, or any other health care provider; nor is it intended to diagnose, treat, cure, or prevent any disease or to be considered medical, psychological, nutritional, or spiritual advice. My intent is not to replace any relationship that exists, or should exist between you and your medical doctor or other health care professional. Always seek the opinion of a physician or other qualified heath care professional regarding any questions or concerns that you might have about your specific health care situation, dietary restrictions, or medications you may be taking. I advise you to speak with your physician before implementing any suggestions about diet, exercise, meditation/ relaxation strategies, or lifestyle; including, but not limited to: taking any supplements, herbal remedies, engaging in any type of cleanse, detox, elimination diet, or modifying any food, exercise, or lifestyle plan. Do not disregard any medical advice that you have received or delay getting medical attention because of any information that you have read in this book. Do not stop taking any medication before speaking with your physician. If you suspect that you have a medical problem, contact your health care provider promptly. Your success depends on your effort and follow-through. I cannot guarantee that you will obtain a particular result, as each individual's success depends on many variables, including, but not limited to your unique health and genetic profile, life history, motivation, and level of commitment.

Table of Contents

Table of Contents Continued

Acknowledgments

I would like to give thanks and praise to my Creator, God, who never fails to provide abundantly. Without His divine grace, I would not have been able to organize my thoughts and put pen to paper. His radiant light, love, peace, and joy are the foundation of my "*glow-rious*" life.

To Olivia, I am truly blessed to have you as my loving daughter. I am thankful for your patience and support during this book writing journey, as well as your technical assistance, which saved my manuscript from extinction on several occasions!

I am grateful for family and friends and their encouragement while writing this book. Deepest gratitude to my friends Nancee, Treva, and Ellen for the time and energy they gave to proofing the first draft.

Sincere appreciation to my editor, Toby, for turning my "writing how I speak" into readable material. A special thank you to my brand specialist, Shari, for not only her help with layout and design, but her encouragement, patience, and sense of humor throughout this endeavor.

I would like to acknowledge and express appreciation to the researchers/authors whose work I internalized and melded into my treatment approach. If I have failed to cite or give credit to anyone, please contact me and I will make the needed adjustments. I am also grateful to my clients for having the courage to share their stories with me and for their trust in trying the *glow approach*. Without the collective wisdom of all of you (clinicians and clients), and the support of my family, friends, and team, there would be no book. I am in deep gratitude to all of you.

Introduction

This workbook is for anyone who has a complicated relationship with food. If you are an emotional or compulsive eater, and you struggle with losing weight and or keeping it off, this workbook is for you. If you are tired of chronic (yo yo) dieting and are wondering if there is an alternative, there is, and it is not another diet.

The glow approach was created to help you change your relationship with food. It is not a diet that you go on or off. It is about developing a healthy relationship with food, which means 1) putting food back in its place — as nutrition (nourishment for your body) and learning what foods "work for you" for health and/or weight-loss; and 2) identifying what role(s) food is playing in your life. For most emotional eaters, food has become a coping mechanism: a way to manage feelings, avoid issues, or fill a void.

You will learn to navigate the bridge between food and feelings, creating awareness and gaining insight into your emotional eating patterns. You will be empowered to listen to your "inner voice" and choose other alternatives to manage your emotions and meet your needs. You will learn to create balance in your life and how to nourish your body • mind • soul • spirit.

If you struggle with food or weight issues, it's not about willpower; it's about creating awareness. The *glow approach* was designed to help you gain insight into what triggers you to eat by exploring the 7 Elements of Transformation: Holistic Nutrition, Emotional Eating, Physiology, Diet Mentality, Modify Your Environment, Healing Body-Image Dissatisfaction, and Sustainable Maintenance; and to create a personalized plan to help you achieve your goals and transform your life.

It's not about the food, yet it is about the food. Making healthful food choices emphasizing nutrient-dense, natural food not only impacts your health, which brings about that outer *glow* (think salmon, avocado, olive oil, leafy greens, etc.), but also, balanced nutrition is essential in reaching and sustaining your weight goals. You will learn what foods "work for you" — not only helping to lose weight and keep it off, but also to feel better physically and mentally.

The inner *glow* is about the other aspects of your life and how fulfilled you are in those areas. The *glow approach* goes beyond balancing calories and the type of food with which you nourish yourself. It's about creating balance in your whole life – balancing relationships, work and play, movement and relaxation, and finding peace in your soul and purpose in your life. It's about loving who you are and who you were meant to be. It's about feeling empowered to take control of your health destiny and living the life you were meant to live. It's about healing your food and weight issues and learning to appreciate the body you have.

Are you ready to begin this journey of transformation?
Are you ready to find your *glow*?

About the *glow approach*

The *glow approach* emerged from my years of clinical work treating clients who were dealing with food and weight issues. Initially, my practice focused on anorexia and bulimia, including patients in a hospital-based eating disorder program.

Eating disorders were considered a biopsychosocial illness and treatment included addressing underlying co-morbidity including personality traits/disorders and other mental-health issues. My doctoral dissertation, written back in 1992, was a treatment plan for eating disordered individuals who had a history of sexual abuse. (Researchers were just beginning to delve into the connection between disordered eating and trauma.)

My practice then evolved to including pre- and post-bariatric surgery psychological consultations. This morphed into referrals from physicians whose patients were struggling with being able to lose weight or keep it off, and cycling from one diet to the next, blaming the diet or themselves for the failure.

I found that most of these "stuck" individuals were emotional eaters and/or they had underlying mental-health issues that were interfering with their weight-loss efforts. If the underlying condition wasn't addressed or treated, the likelihood for relapse was probable. My Emotional Eating and Physiology chapters highlight these insights.

Although addressing the client's emotional eating and treating the condition that was being "self-medicated" significantly decreased the non-hunger eating, I noted that there were still other elements that would trigger eating or overeating, including environmental food cues (Modify Your Environment) and negative thoughts or self-talk (Diet Mentality).

As a former RN I have always had a passion for health, wellness, and nutrition. This passion increased to an even higher level after I completed my health coach training, which modernized my view of food. I incorporate this perspective into my Holistic Nutrition chapter.

I have always told my clients that losing weight and keeping it off is not an easy journey. There are many pieces to the puzzle and each element has to be addressed. I believe that as an individual becomes more comfortable in their own skin, the obsessing with dieting decreases and a more realistic lifestyle approach to weight-loss is possible. I address this in my Healing Body-Image Dissatisfaction chapter.

Some people are successful in taking the weight off, but time and again, eventually regain the weight. We are creatures of habit, convenience, and pavlovian response. We are bombarded by subliminal dichotomous marketing, "supersize your food, but downsize your body." Food serves an emotional purpose and weight (body size) may too. I explore these and other possible reasons for relapse in my last chapter Sustainable Maintenance.

I am honored to be your guide as you begin your journey of transformation.

Get the *glow*!

Chapter 1 Summary

- The Role of Food – Nourishing Your Body
- Individualized Approach – Biopsychosocial Uniqueness
- Goal Setting and Increasing Motivation
- Eat Empowered
    - Eat without Shame or Guilt
    - Eat with Respect for Your Body's Needs
    - Eat with Body Awareness
    - Eat Mindfully
- Mindful Eating Exercise
- Internal Cues for Hunger and Satiety
- Balanced Nutrition
- Balance Strategies
    - Tier Approach
    - Planning and Compensating
- Foods that Help with or Inhibit Weight-Loss
- Managing Food Cravings
    - How to Eat Highly Desired Foods

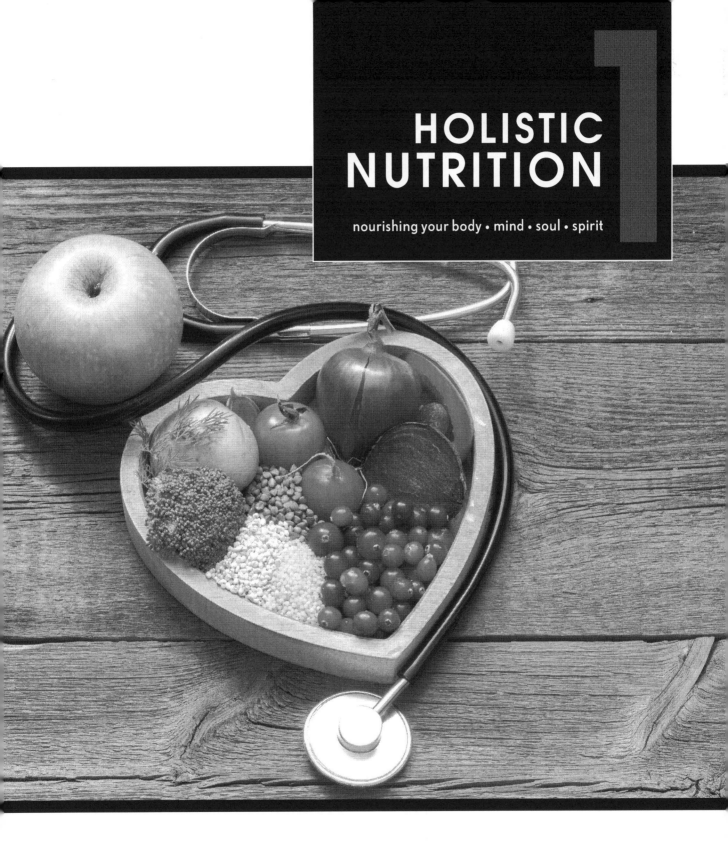

HOLISTIC NUTRITION

1

nourishing your body • mind • soul • spirit

"They will be radiant because of the many gifts the Lord has given them— the abundant crops of grain, new wine and olive oil." – Jeremiah 31:12

glow's approach to nutrition focuses on getting food back into the leading role it was meant to be in: nourishment for your mind and body. This requires a significant change in mindset, which will greatly improve your ability to make healthier choices in what you feed your body **and** to follow through with lifestyle changes.

Nutrient-dense whole foods are a key element in reaching and sustaining weight loss goals as well as improving overall physical and mental health. As Hippocrates stated, "Let food be thy medicine."

What we put into our body can help, hurt, or heal us. Instead of viewing food as just good or bad, we need to begin to look at it as nourishment and fuel for our body. What we eat becomes our blood, our cells, our organs, our brain, and therefore, impacts not only our physical health, but our mental health as well (Rosenthol, 2015).

Focus On Your Health, Not "Dieting"

Do you want to lose weight **and** be healthy too? Nutrient-dense whole foods program the body to function properly and promote optimal health. Nutrigenomics is the scientific study of the interaction of nutrition and genes, especially with regard to the prevention or treatment of disease, including obesity. Dr. Mark Hyman, MD, a well-known functional medicine physician, writes about this in his book, *The Blood Sugar Solution*, "Food is information and it controls your gene expression, hormones, and metabolism." (p. 194)

Dr. Hyman's (2012) plan to control "diabesity" focuses on foods that are anti-inflammatory and stabilize blood-sugar. This includes low glycemic-load vegetables and seaweed, whole grains, legumes, and low glycemic-load fruits in moderation. It also limits high glycemic-load vegetables and fruits. Processed foods are avoided, as well as flour products and sugar in any form. Gluten and dairy (two major inflammatory foods) are avoided in the jumpstart part of the program, and may or may not be reintroduced depending on how your body responds to them.[1]

We now know that cellular inflammation is linked to the most commonly occurring diseases including **obesity**, diabetes, heart disease, cancer, Alzheimer's, depression, arthritis, and other disorders, including auto-immune diseases and allergies.

Dr. Hyman's, *The Blood Sugar Solution* is an excellent resource on how to locate the causes of inflammation in your body and eliminate them.

---

[1] From *The Blood Sugar Solution* by Mark Hyman, M.D., copyright © 2012. Reprinted by permission of Little, Brown, and Company, an imprint of Hachette Book Group, Inc.

"Sugar, refined carbohydrates, trans fats, too many omega-6 fats from processed plant oils (such as soybean or corn oil), artificial sweeteners, hidden food allergies and sensitivities, chronic infections, imbalances in gut bacteria, environmental toxins, stress, and a sedentary lifestyle all contribute to inflammation." (p. 99)

If you are currently struggling with a medical or mental health condition that is associated with inflammation, Dr. Don Colbert MD's, *Let Food Be Your Medicine*, outlines a modified Mediterranean diet that can prevent or reverse disease, including obesity. Each chapter discusses a specific disorder and what foods to eat more or less of, with a modified Mediterranean diet as the foundation.

The Mediterranean diet was known as one of the best anti-inflammatory diets, but results began to decline, especially in the United States. Dr. Colbert, along with Dr. William Davis, *Wheat Belly*, and Dr. David Perlmutter, *Grain Brain*, propose that wheat and corn are not the same as they use to be; most have been genetically modified, which can contribute to inflammation. Thus, Dr. Colbert's modifications eliminate or greatly limit gluten and corn as well as avoid or limit other GMO foods (soy, cottonseed and canola oil, sugar beets, and papaya). His plan emphasizes a mostly plant-based diet, with healthy fats (including wild salmon), low-glycemic index starches, and limits red meat, dairy, and eggs.

Another leading expert in the field of obesity, Dr. David Ludwig, *Always Hungry*, designed his program to lower body-weight set point by targeting insulin resistance and chronic inflammation through improving food and sleep quality, decreasing stress, and increasing activity level. His plan focuses on how food affects our bodies and ultimately our fat cells. The types of calories we eat affect the number of calories we burn. Highly processed carbohydrates digest rapidly and raise blood sugar and program our fat cells to hoard calories.

Stress, sleep deprivation, and sedentary habits also force cells into calorie-storage overdrive, which Debra Waterhouse, MPH, RD also sites, almost 30 years ago in her ground-breaking books, *Outsmarting the Female Fat Cell*, and *Outsmarting the Midlife Fat Cell*. She also includes the following as activating the lipogenic (fat storing) enzyme: skipping meals, overeating, night eating, and estrogen (puberty, pregnancy, BCP, estrogen replacement, and menopause).

There are many diets and food plans that focus on "burning fat" by consuming a high protein, low carbohydrate diet, including Eco-Atkins, South Beach, Zone, Paleo, and others. Most of these plans focus on low-glycemic carbohydrates, healthy fats, and healthy or plant- based proteins. Dr. Ludwig also recommends low-glycemic carbohydrates, but in phase one, (jump start) of his "always hungry solution," he starts out with 50% fat, mostly unsaturated, but also includes full fat dairy, coconut, and chocolate. Participants report less hunger, fewer cravings, and improved energy and mood on this highly satiating food plan.

The majority of functional medicine providers advise increasing the quality of the food we eat by eating "clean" which includes eating whole, natural food and buying seasonal and organic when you can (especially the dirty dozen). Shop for animal products that are pasture-raised, grass-fed and antibiotic-, hormone- and pesticide-free. Buy wild or sustainably farmed fish. Eliminating high fructose corn syrup and trans fats are also recommended.

Joshua Rosenthal, founder and director of the Institute for Integrative Nutrition, has researched over 100 different dietary theories. His philosophy is that because of our bioindividuality, one diet can not fit everyone and you need to find the fit that is right for you. Joshua (2014) has summarized a food plan that focuses on "adding in" and "crowding out".

> *"Focus on adding in whole organic foods. Diet is plant-centered, especially green vegetables and seaweed, fruit, seeds and nuts, healthy oils, non-GMO whole grains and legumes. Grass-fed beef and free-range chickens/eggs without hormones and antibiotics are also suggested. Joshua also recommends increasing water intake, being more active, and cooking at home. Crowd out sugar, refined carbohydrates, processed foods, partially hydrogenated oils, red meat, dairy, alcohol "liquid sugar," caffeine, salt, chemicals, preservatives, artificial sweeteners, high fructose corn syrup, and fast food."*

Joshua also discusses lifestyle factors, "primary foods" that create optimal health: relationships, physical activity, career, and spirituality. Blue Zone author and researcher, Dan Buettner (2008) also sites lifestyle choices as being instrumental in influencing health and well-being in the individuals who live in the different areas of the world that live longer and have better quality of life. The 10 main Blue Zone food guidelines also focus on plant based whole foods, eating healthy fish 3x/week, enjoying 1 cup of beans and a handful of nuts per day, limiting meat and dairy, limiting sugar to < 7 tsp/day, and limiting whole grain (sourdough bread is acceptable). As for beverages, drink mostly water; tea and coffee are allowed, as well as a limited amount of wine.

The glow Approach Helps You Discover What Food Plan Works Best for YOU

There are many food plans and diets to choose from. Ultimately, the one that is going to work for you is one that you can maintain long-term, and is a fit for you. As a health coach, I chose to highlight other professionals' food plans because of their focus on health. Healthful eating typically has weight loss as an indirect benefit.

Understanding your biopsychosocial uniqueness is vital in helping you identify what **you** need to do to achieve **and** maintain success (health goals and/or weight-loss). (The term biopsychosocial uniqueness was inspired in part by Joshua Rosenthal's, *Institute of Integrative Nutrition* "bioindividuality"™ and the study of eating disorders from a biopsychosocial perspective.)

At *glow*, the **first step** in the process is your biopsychosocial assessment *(see Appendix A)* which includes but is not limited to your food/weight history, food preferences, food intolerances, lifestyle, culture/religion, personality traits, mental and emotional health, medical and health conditions, family history, cooking style, budget, and time. You will use this information to guide you in designing a plan that is unique to you. You decide what is on your plan by listening to your body and how food affects you, and by what your health and weight goals are. Your personalized plan, combined with *the glow approach* will give you what you need to have optimal success.

These nutritional and lifestyle changes need to be gradual and sustainable, and they need to address who you are and what your body needs. Once you decide what your goals are, you can choose which plan you want to begin with. (Please consult with your healthcare professional before beginning any dietary or exercise plan or making other lifestyle changes.)

If you have an active eating disorder, eating stabilization is typically the first phase, and a non-restrictive approach to weight-loss/maintenance is advised. "Dieting", especially if it eliminates food groups or has too many restrictions, is contraindicated for individuals who struggle with bulimia or binge-eating disorder. It is highly recommended that you also work with a professional who specializes in eating disorders.

Let's Get Started!

You need to have a purpose and a strategy for whatever your goal is. Goals reflect what you value. Goal setting gives you focus and clarity, helps you to prioritize and organize your time, and motivates you to take responsibility for the personal growth and change you want in your life.

Define your Goal: (i.e., weight loss, end emotional eating, eliminate symptoms, or other)

_____

_____

Set SMART Goals:

Specific _____

_____

Measurable _____

_____

Attainable _____

_____

Realistic _____

_____

Time-Limited _____

_____

When determining attainable and realistic, especially with weight and body shape, take into account some of the physiological realities of your life including age and stage of life, i.e., perimenopause and post-menopause, metabolic conditions, etc. *(See Physiology and Body-Image chapters.)*

Next is **"The Big Why?"** That is the key to your motivation. Think about all of the different reasons including what you will gain and what you will eliminate by making the changes.

_____

_____

Short-Term or External Motivators (These may help you kick-start your program but may not be enough to maintain it. *i.e., appearance or 25-year class reunion*)

_____

_____

Long-Term or Internal Motivators (These keep you on track for the long-haul. *i.e., health, being alive for kids or grandkids*)

_____

_____

How: What plan has worked for you best in the past? _____

_____

_____

What made it difficult to stick to? _____

_____

_____

What were the pros and cons of various plans you have used? Is there a way to combine the best of the best and leave out the rest? If it is a restrictive plan, does it work for you emotionally or does it trigger a rebound "all or none" eating style? Is there a way to modify the plan or to have it as a time-limited phase?

_____

_____

_____

Timing: Why now? _____

_____

_____

Is this a good time for you to take on making lifestyle changes? Is there anything else going on in your life that might be a distraction? _____

_____

_____

If you are currently experiencing a major life stressor, focusing on healthful eating and weight maintenance, as well as self-care strategies may be all that you have the energy for. That's totally okay; you can skip to those sections now. And when you feel ready (have the focus and energy) to begin transforming your life–jump back in!

glow's Maintenance Plan

Eat Empowered

You have choices! Don't give your power away! You can change, grow, and transform!

- Eat without Guilt or Shame
- Eat with Respect for Your Body's Needs
- Eat with Body Awareness (How food makes you feel physically)
- Eat Mindfully

Eat Without Guilt or Shame

Eating is not a moral issue. We make it one. We let it determine our worth, our mood, our involvement in social activities or relationships. Stop judging yourself by what you eat. You don't have to feel bad about eating or your weight—you deserve to eat!

You don't have to feel shame about your eating behavior—**Food Works!** If you are eating or overeating for emotional reasons, you will learn how food works on many different levels. Physiologically it works on your neurotransmitters and hormones. It relaxes, suppresses, numbs-out, or gives you a lift. It's a sensual pleasure. It provides structure or a way to defocus or avoid what you are feeling. Your body is trying to take care of you on some level, and by **eating with awareness**, you will begin to see the different roles food serves in your life. *(See Emotional Eating chapter.)*

Enjoy the food you love without the guilt, and it will lose its power over you. The obsession will decrease. It is okay to eat for pleasure as long as you are getting this need met in other areas of your life as well.

Instead of labeling foods as good or bad, which then may lead to how you feel about yourself, look at the food from a nutrition perspective. Some foods are more healthful, others are empty calories, and some actually contribute to disease.

Eat with Respect for Your Body's Needs

Change your focus from a diet-mentality to a health and wellness approach. Instead of feeling deprived and obsessing about what you cannot eat because you are on a diet, focus on what you need to eat to nourish your body and be mindful of how the food makes you feel physically and mentally. Your self-talk will change from, "what I can't have" to "what does my body need." As you focus on including more healthful options, there is less room for unhealthy food.

What foods do I need to nourish my body? (What are my health conditions, food sensitivities, family history, etc.?) _____

_____

_____

_____

What does this food do for my body? What are the nutrients and micronutrients in this food, and how do they impact my physical and mental health? _____

_____

_____

_____

Eat with Body Awareness

When you are choosing a food to eat, instead of feeling deprived. i.e., "I can't have this because I am dieting" focus on, "How does this food make me feel physically and/or mentally?"

What changes do you notice in your mind/body after you eat this food? How does this impact your energy level, mental alertness/brain fog, inflammation or pain, skin conditions, respiratory/cardiac systems, or gastrointestinal symptoms including diarrhea, constipation, bloating, reflux, or pain?

_____

_____

_____

When you focus on what nutrients your body needs and how food makes your body feel, you will begin to make healthier choices on what you put into your body.

Eat Mindfully

This strategy evolved from the practice of mindfulness—focusing one's awareness on the present moment while noticing, without judgment, thoughts, feelings, and bodily sensations. Mindful eating helps you to focus on **eating with awareness** to taste and using all of your senses to satisfy "mouth hunger," as well as being aware of hunger and satiety cues.

"Intuitive Eating," as defined by Evelyn Tribole, MS, RD and Elyse Resch, MS, RD, in their groundbreaking book, *Intuitive Eating: A Revolutionary Program that Works*, includes the principles of mindful eating, unconditional permission to eat when hungry and to eat the food that is desired. It also addresses cognition, emotions, and body-image.

Although many diet plans have you monitor your food intake, Linda Craighead, PhD, *The Appetite Awareness Workbook*, has you monitor your appetite. Her program, Appetite Awareness Training, utilizes mindfulness and the role of internal cues to determine hunger and satiety. AAT teaches you to use stomach fullness instead of feelings of satisfaction to decide when to stop eating.

The glow approach will help you recognize internal cues for hunger and satiety, rather than eating or overeating when you are cued by non-hunger triggers. You will learn to be mindful on all levels: eating when physically hungry, stopping when comfortably full, and enjoying food without feeling guilty.

Mindful Eating

Jon Kabat Zinn (1990), a pioneer in the mindfulness movement, illustrates the concept of mindful eating with his "raisin meditation." He guides you in using all of your senses, one after another, to observe a raisin in great detail, from the way it feels in your hand to the way its taste bursts on your tongue. This exercise is intended to help you focus on the present moment, and can be tried with other foods, and even your entire dining experience.

Mindful Eating Experience *(Reconnecting with your Hunger and Satiety Cues)*

1. Prepare a meal that has a combination of healthy fats, carbohydrates, and proteins using a variety of temperatures, textures, colors, and flavors. Include a 16-oz. glass of cold water, with or without lemon.

2. Turn on relaxing background music. Light a candle.

3. Close your eyes and relax. Notice any feelings you are having.

4. Be aware of your breathing. Take slow, slightly deep breaths.

5. Open your eyes and look at your food. Be aware of the colors, textures, and aroma.

6. Be aware of your level of hunger.

7. Take a drink of your liquid.

8. Take a bite and begin to eat. Be aware of chewing and swallowing.

9. Put only small bites on your fork and be sure to put your fork down between bites.

10. Chew your food completely. Move the food around in your mouth to alleviate "mouth hunger." Notice the texture, temperature, and flavor.

11. Notice what you like and do not like.

12. Notice if there are any feelings coming up for you as you are eating.

13. Return your focus to your breathing.

14. Resume eating. Take a drink of your beverage when you want to.

15. After 10 minutes, notice your level of hunger or fullness. This is the half-way mark to the 20 minutes it takes for your blood sugar to rise and your appestat (satiety center) in your brain to signal your stomach that you are full.

16. Continue eating, noticing how the food tastes. Take a drink when you want to.

17. At 20 minutes, notice your level of fullness. Learn to distinguish between comfortably full and stuffed.

18. You may drink more of your beverage if you wish. This can signal that you are done with your meal.

What did you notice or learn about yourself?_____

_____

_____

_____

_____

Use this strategy any time you need to eat mindfully – to alleviate "mouth hunger," and/ or when you want to reconnect with internal cues for hunger and satiety. You can also do a mini version of this exercise, substituting an orange. Utilize all of your senses to truly capture the essence of this experience.

Rating Hunger/Fullness

It is often helpful to use some type of a rating scale for appetite awareness to help monitor internal cues. This is just one example. You can modify it to fit you. (1-10)

1. Extreme hunger, dizziness
2. Very hungry, irritable
3. Strong signals to eat
4. First sign that your body needs food, stomach rumble (3-4 hours after last meal)
5. Partially full
6. Comfortably full, satisfied
7. Slightly over-full
8. Starting to feel uncomfortable
9. Very full and bloated
10. So full that it hurts, stuffed, nauseas

The Key to Long-Term Success is Balance

glow is about balance. One food, one meal, one day won't make or break your health or your weight-loss goal. It is the patterns of food choices that will determine the outcome, so you still need to be mindful of the truth of what you are putting into your body and have the awareness of choice, options, and consequences.

Be mindful of what you are eating and take responsibility for food choices. We obviously need to look at the quality of food we are giving our bodies, and our perspective should change. Instead of thinking, "This is fattening," replace the thought with, "How is this food impacting my health, and how does it make me feel physically and mentally?"

24

Most foods can fit into a **balanced** diet using moderation, variety, and being mindful when eating high-risk foods. Moderation may mean decreasing the amount and frequency of unhealthy food, but not necessarily eliminating it. Too much restriction can set you up for failure. Limiting calories or food groups can trigger cravings, hunger, and "all or none" diet mentality, as well as putting you at risk for bingeing. Elimination of a food may come later as a choice based on internal cues (i.e., health concerns, physical response to the food, or food addiction strategies), not diet mentality.

You don't need to be perfect to reach your goal; an 80/20 ratio may be more attainable.

Balancing Your Body's Needs

Food is made up of three main macronutrients (protein, carbohydrates, and fat). Understanding how each function in the body will help guide your decision making with your food plan, as well as give you factual information to challenge diet mentality.

Carbohydrates

Carbohydrates give us energy and are full of vitamins, minerals, phytonutrients, and fiber. They are precursors to neurotransmitters that help regulate our mood and other bodily functions.

Fats

Our body needs dietary fats for the absorption of Vitamins A, D, E, and K. Fats are building blocks for our hormones that regulate bodily functions. Our immune system requires fats to function properly. Our nerves are coated with fatty insulation. Our eyes need healthy fat for good vision since the retina is actually a layer of nerves. Our brain is 60% fat, so healthy fats improve thinking and help prevent depression and moodiness.

Protein

Protein helps build new blood, tissue, and bone cells, as well as build and repair muscle. It helps keep your heart healthy, since your heart is a muscle. It combines with iron to form hemoglobin in the blood. It is a precursor to hormones and enzymes. It helps build antibodies with which the body fights infection, and it helps to balance blood sugar and metabolism.

Fiber

The benefits of increasing fiber include: lowering cholesterol, helping fight heart disease, reducing risk of certain cancers, helping control blood sugar levels, and helping prevent constipation. It also creates a sense of fullness so you don't overeat, and it keeps you full longer.

What Does a Typical Food Plan Look Like?

You can aim for a macronutrient (protein, fat, carbohydrates) percentage depending on your health and or weight goals. Your "plate" will divide up accordingly. Specific food choices will also depend on which micronutrients (vitamins and minerals) and phytonutrients (found in plants - flavonoids, resveratrol, carotenoids, polyphenols, etc.) you want to nourish your body with.

- Typical weight-loss percentage: 30% protein, 30% fat, 40% carbohydrates.
- Typical health promoting/anti-inflammatory percentage (based on the Mediterranean Diet): 16% protein, 38% fat, 46% carbohydrates.

   Plant-based protein is the focus, with fish and some poultry, limited red meat and dairy, and includes monosaturated fats and whole grains. The modified version avoids gluten and corn.

How to Fill Your Plate

Greens and Low-Carbohydrate Vegetables (1/2 of your plate)

Spinach, kale, Swiss chard, cabbage, bok choy, romaine lettuce, broccoli, cauliflower, brussel sprouts, asparagus, green beans, tomatoes, cucumber, celery, onion, garlic, peppers, radishes, summer squash, mushrooms, etc.

Protein (1/4 of your plate)

Plant based proteins count, too! Beans, peas, lentils, nuts and nut butters, seeds, etc. Lean protein including wild fish, poultry, eggs, and red meat in moderation.

Healthy Carbohydrates (Starchy) (1/8 of your plate)

Whole grains including brown rice, quinoa, steel cut oatmeal, and corn have moderate glycemic index/glycemic load (GI/GL). Winter squash, carrots, peas, beets, beans, and lentils have moderate GI, but have a low GL. Sweet potatoes have a high GI/GL.

Healthy Fat (1/8 of your plate)

Olive oil, walnut oil, coconut oil (in moderation), salmon, avocados, olives, nuts and nut butters, seeds including flax and chia, 70% dark chocolate (in moderation).

Fruit

Counts as a carbohydrate. Most fruits have a low GL because they are high in fiber. Limit dried fruit and fruit juice (high GI).

Dairy (Optional)

Can count towards protein, carbohydrates, and fat.

Portion Control

Be mindful of serving size. Use visual cues. Calories are estimates. It is okay to estimate so you do not become obsessed with calorie counting.

Vegetables: ½ cup cooked or 1 c. raw (baseball sized) = 25 calories, leafy greens: 2 c. (2 baseballs) = 25 cal.

Fruit: ½ c. sliced or medium piece (baseball) = 50-100 cal.

Carbohydrates: ½ c. rice, pasta (hockey puck) = 75 cal.; ½ c. beans = 125 cal., ½ c. corn/ peas/sweet potato = 90 cal.; ½ c. winter squash/pumpkin = 40 cal.

Protein/Dairy: 3 oz. fish, 2-3 oz meat (deck of cards) = 100 - 200 cal., 1 oz. or ¼ c. shredded cheese (1/3 deck of cards) = 100 cal.

Fats: 100 cal. = 1 tbsp peanut butter, 1/3 medium avocado, 2 ½ tsp olive oil, 10-15 nuts, 2 tbsp seeds.

Fiber: 25-35 gms/day. Beans are one of the best sources of fiber: 1/2c., lentils = 8gms, ½ c. chick peas = 6 gms; nuts and seeds = 2-4 gms/ serving; 1 cup of avocado = 10gms, ½ grapefruit = 6 gms, 1 c. raspberries = 8 gms; 1 c. bran cereal = 20 gms, 1 c. oatmeal = 4 gms.

Snacks: Think of a snack as a mini-meal. Aim for a protein/fiber combination. Use snacks to help keep blood sugar balanced and to prevent overeating at the next meal. Think of sugar, refined carbohydrates, sweets, etc. as treats. Snacks are a scheduled part of your food plan. Treats should be occasional, but can be scheduled as well so you can plan and compensate for them.

glow's Balance Strategies

How to Find Balance

Balance eating for nutrition (to nourish your body) with eating for pleasure (enjoying the food you eat). Be aware of how much of and how often you are eating certain foods (like treats) and the impact it is having on your health and weight goals.

Some people like to keep track by counting calories, others use food groups, exchanges, serving size, or points. Some people are in tune with their internal cues for hunger/satiety and stop eating when they are comfortably full. The first approach is more structured; the second is more intuitive.

The Tier Approach

This strategy is easily explained using calories, but you can also substitute exchanges, points, or food groups.

> *Example: If your calorie limit for weight-loss is 1500 per day (which would result in a healthy and realistic 2 pound per week weight-loss, depending on your current weight and activity level) instead of holding to that one number and being fearful of going over, set up a tier of ranges to allow for flexibility, not only during the weight-loss stage but also during maintenance.*

Pre-Tier: Ketogenic Diets

1st Tier: 1400-1600 Weight-Loss

2nd Tier: 1600-1800 Slow Weight-Loss

3rd Tier: 1800-2000 Maintenance

Please note that the above calorie amounts are arbitrary. Specific guidelines are based on gender, height, weight, and lifestyle activity (sedentary to very active).

Examples of How to Use the Tier Approach:

• Your goal is to lose 2 lbs. per week. You start the day by aiming for the 1st tier. You get invited to dinner. Instead of declining or overeating, you aim for the 2nd or 3rd tier. You are still in the process of weight loss, even though it will be slightly less, or the day may end up being a maintenance day. In the long run, you will be able to stay on your plan because of the flexibility it affords you.

- You are in weight-loss mode. You are planning to go on vacation for a week. The week before the trip you aim for the 1st tier every day. (Pre-trip weight loss of 2#). While on the trip you aim for the 3rd tier. (Focusing on maintenance during the trip may help you avoid overeating and at the same time help you feel like you are not depriving yourself). You could have an average weight loss of a pound over those two weeks. Or if you overindulge on the trip, your weight stays the same over the two-week period.

Planning and Compensating

This strategy helps you balance your calories and nutrition. Learn to plan or compensate for a treat, a calorie dense food, or empty calorie food. This could be within a meal, within the day, or within the week. This can be used with holidays, vacations, restaurant eating, etc.

Examples of How to Use Planning and Compensating:

- **Planning:** You have plans to go out to dinner. For breakfast and lunch choose healthy lower calorie, nutrient-dense foods, focusing on lean protein, healthy fat, and healthy carbohydrates (vegetables, fruit, etc.).
- **Planning:** If you are going out of town for the weekend, plan to be on 1st tier Monday through Thursday, so you can bank calories for the weekend.
- **Compensating:** You eat a typical breakfast, but then your boss brings in Mexican food for lunch. You can even stay within the 1st tier for the day if you compensate at dinner with a lower calorie, nutrient-dense meal (grilled chicken breast, 2 servings of vegetables or leafy greens).

Your *glow* Plan

As discussed earlier, most plans start with a "jump-start" phase. I would like to encourage you to look at this "jump-start" period as time-limited and focused on health, healing, and self-discovery. *glow* is about helping you to choose foods that work for you.

What are your food/weight/health goals? _____

_____

_____

_____

_____

This may be a good time to reboot your system. Depending on your needs and your biopsychosocial uniqueness, you decide what your Reboot looks like.

Reboot

- **Renew**: Detox or Cleanse (very time-limited)
- **Restore:**
  1. *Elimination Diet:* Assessing for food allergies/sensitivities and/or healing your microbiome.
  2. *Specific Diet for Medical Condition:* i.e., FODMAP for bloating and other GI symptoms or Body Ecology diet for Candida, IBS, or "leaky gut."
- **Rebalance:** "Clean eating." The focus is on nutrient-dense, natural food. Eliminate or avoid sugar, refined carbohydrates, and/or other (coffee or other forms of caffeine, alcohol, gluten, dairy, soy, etc.) if you choose.

Food Choices for Health, Satiety, and Satisfaction

glow's philosophy regarding nutrition is to make food work for you. The right food can improve health, decrease inflammation, increase energy, and even give your skin that healthy glow. You will learn which food will fill you up and keep you full, as well as satisfy cravings. Although you will design a plan that is unique to you, there are still fundamental guidelines that are beneficial for most individuals.

Increase or Add:

- Water
- Nutrient-dense whole food: Leafy greens and other vegetable, fruit, legumes (lentils, peas and, beans, peanuts, and carob), nuts and seeds, healthy fats (olive oil, avocado, salmon), whole grains, plant based and lean proteins.
- Super-foods *(See Appendix B.)*
- Fiber

Decrease or Eliminate: sugar (including high-fructose corn syrup), refined carbohydrates, processed foods, nitrates, trans-fats, and partially hydrogenated oils.

Monitor: red meat, dairy, gluten, soy, salt (explore the pros/cons of these for your body, i.e. allergies, food sensitivities, health conditions). Other high allergy-potential foods include peanuts, nuts, shellfish, eggs, citrus, night shade vegetables, corn, yeast, MSG, artificial color/flavor/sweeteners, GMOs, and alcohol. Be mindful of coffee, caffeine intake, and its impact on your body (coffee stimulates stomach acid which can lead to inflammation).

Be mindful about alcohol use. Alcohol is liquid sugar, so not only does it decrease inhibitions and trigger over-eating; it also leads to carbohydrate cravings the next day. In addition, alcohol kills friendly bacteria in the digestive tract.

Buy organic, seasonal, and local when you can. Be aware of the clean 15/dirty dozen produce. Look for grass-fed, free-range, antibiotic and hormone-free protein and dairy. Plant a garden, cook at home, and know where your food comes from.

glow's Weight-Loss Plan

Create Awareness and gain insight into what is triggering you to eat by exploring the 7 Elements of Transformation and utilizing your Awareness Record. When you learn to differentiate physical hunger from emotional eating and other non-hunger cues, you have the opportunity to not use food in that role and instead, replace it with a new pattern. This strategy alone may be enough for you to eliminate compulsive eating and release unwanted pounds.

You will not see a specific "typical diet" food plan as a core element in this workbook. You will be designing a plan that fits your biopsychosocial uniqueness. No one will tell you what to eat. It will be you listening to your body. I will give you suggestions and provide you with the latest research, but ultimately you get to decide what fits and works for you.

Your weight-loss plan should look as close as possible to your maintenance plan, ensuring a smoother transition once you reach your goal weight. The Tier-Approach is one concept I use to help facilitate this philosophy. During the weight-loss phase, you will want to be mindful of choosing foods that "work" for you (fill you up and keep you full, decrease cravings, and burn fat).

The "Best" Weight-Loss Foods (Making Food Work for You)

Fill You Up and Keep You Full *(See Appendix B for superfoods that may assist with weight-loss.)*

Volume

- Water before or with meals (16 oz.) or broth based soup

High Fiber: legumes, whole grains, vegetables, fruit

- Fiber slows the passage of food through your digestive tract, making you feel full longer. It also plays a role in keeping blood sugar stable, thus decreasing food cravings. Fiber and liquid stretch the stomach walls which decreases ghrelin (hunger stimulating hormone).

Food That You Have to Chew: salads, vegetables, protein.

- It takes 20 minutes for your brain to signal your stomach that you are full. Slow down your rate of eating.

Protein (including plant-based) and **Healthy Fat:** nuts, seeds, avocado, olive oil, etc.

- Protein and fat take longer to pass through your digestive tract, making you feel full longer (satiety). Healthy fat can decrease cravings for sugar and refined carbohydrates.

Fiber-Rich Low-Starch Carbohydrates: vegetables and legumes.

- Fewer calories are absorbed if raw or high fiber.

Stop Filling Your Stomach When it is 4/5 Full to Help Aid Digestion

- Be mindful of portion size.

Foods that Inhibit Weight-Loss: Sugar and Refined Carbohydrates

This is from a Health Perspective:

- Sugar and refined carbohydrates cause inflammation.
- Cellular inflammation is linked to obesity, diabetes, heart disease, cancer, Alzheimer's, arthritis, and other disorders, including auto-immune diseases.

Understanding How Sugar Affects Blood Sugar:

- **Insulin:** a hormone that "unlocks" cells to move blood sugar (glucose) into cells where it can be used as fuel.
- **Insulin Resistance:** cells are no longer responding to insulin.

Weight gain and visceral fat can bring on insulin resistance by producing inflammatory chemicals that harm the cell so the cell can no longer take glucose from the blood. This results in high blood sugar. High blood sugar over time can lead to diabetes.

- High blood sugar signals the release of insulin, which tells the body to store extra sugar as fat.

- Eating sugar and refined carbohydrates increases blood sugar, which causes inflammation, which in turn increases risk of disease.

High-glycemic carbohydrates create a large, temporary increase in blood sugar because they digest quickly so more insulin is released. The insulin instructs the body to store the calories as fat, then closes the cellular "door," which restricts the ability of those calories to get out. A decrease in the blood glucose and lipids then occurs.

Thus, the result is low blood sugar which triggers hunger and cravings for a quick fix, i.e., sugar and refined carbohydrates. This also will trigger the brain to decrease metabolism and inhibit the release of glycogen, which instructs the body to burn stored fat.

Glycemic Index and Glycemic Load

The glycemic index (GI) is a value assigned to a food based on how quickly that food causes an increase in blood sugar levels. Foods low on the GI tend to release glucose slowly, keep blood sugars steady, and foster weight-loss. Foods high on the GI scale release glucose rapidly, which helps with energy recovery after exercise, but is not healthy for individuals with pre-diabetes/diabetes or who are trying to manage their weight. A GI <55 is low, medium is 56-69, 70+ is high.

To understand a food's complete effect on blood sugar, you need to know how quickly the food makes glucose enter the blood stream and how much glucose it will deliver. The glycemic load (GL) tells how much glucose a food will deliver, which gives a more accurate picture of a food's impact on blood sugar. GL = GI x grams of carbohydrates in a serving, then divide by 10. A GL of 10 or below is considered low; 20 or above is considered high. (Harvard Medical School, 2015)

What Can You Do? *Eat with Awareness*

When you decrease your sugar and refined carbohydrate intake, less insulin is needed. You are taking control of reprogramming your fat cells to release stored glucose and lipids, which are used as fuel, resulting in decreased hunger and stabilized metabolism. This is a natural way to readjust your body-weight set point.

- Decrease visceral (belly) fat by increasing fiber, monosaturated fats, and whole grains.

- Balance protein, healthy fats, and fiber (which slows digestion).

- Eat (healthy) carbohydrates at the end of meal to minimize the rise in blood sugar and insulin. If the carbohydrate is a snack, pair it with protein or fiber.

- Eat small portions 6x/day to keep blood sugar steady (if this works for you) or have your largest meal at breakfast or lunch and your smallest meal at dinnertime.

- Add M&M's . . . movement and meditation! *(See Physiology chapter.)*

> **Movement (Exercise):** Helps muscles take in glucose without need for insulin, so you are burning the sugar as fuel and it won't be stored as fat.

> **Meditation (Relaxation):** Stress triggers our fight and flight response, which instructs our cells to release sugar for fuel, but at the same time, inhibits the release of insulin because our body thinks we need the fuel to fight or run from danger. Since most of our stress today is psychological, the sugar lingers in our blood stream but eventually is stored as fat.

Most "diets" work to a degree because they eliminate junk food. Thus, it should not be a surprise that most of the health-promoting diets begin with a 2-week jumpstart that eliminates certain foods and beverages. Lowering your carbohydrate intake is the quickest and easiest way to decrease insulin levels and jumpstart weight-loss. Limit sugar and refined carbohydrates. When you do eat carbohydrates, choose healthy carbohydrates, including whole grains, fruit, starchy vegetables, legumes in moderation, and unlimited amounts of low-glycemic load vegetables.

In regard to balancing carbohydrates, some individuals do better with high protein/low carbohydrate meals at breakfast and lunch and including carbohydrates with the evening meal. This approach limits the sugar/insulin dynamic and may help you feel full on fewer calories. Other individuals feel that they do better with some amount of carbohydrates at every meal. "Do better" could mean – feeling full longer, feeling more satisfied, having less cravings, etc. Remember, your plan is the one that works for you.

Weight-loss food plans are meant to be time-limited. Even if you have not reached your weight goal, you may benefit from taking a break and allowing yourself to be on the "maintenance tier" for a while. This actually can give you a little boost in your metabolism and allows you more flexibility with food options.

Taking a break can actually help you renew your energy and motivation to continue with your weight-loss goals. The key is to continue with "Balance" concepts (plan/compensate, tier approach, and plan B) and not resort to all/none eating style (unhealthy food choices, overeating, etc.).

Learn How to Eat, Not Overeat

Understanding and Managing Your Food Cravings:

1. Utilize *glow's* Awareness Record to first eliminate non-hunger food cues. It may not be food that you are craving.

2. Try drinking a low or non-caloric beverage – you may actually be thirsty.

3. Try getting sweet flavor earlier in the day. Fruit, starchy or roasted vegetables, and nut butters are some healthy options.

4. Have a balance of healthy carbohydrates, healthy fats, and healthy protein at each meal.

5. Snacks should contain protein and fiber.

6. Healthy fat can shut off craving center in the brain.

7. Have a high protein breakfast.

8. Eat your larger meal earlier in the day.

9. If you are drinking your calories or are eating a high sugar/refined carbohydrate snack or meal, be prepared for a blood sugar spike and crash, followed by carbohydrate cravings.

10. If you are eating or drinking "diet" food, the artificial sweeteners may trick your pancreas into thinking it needs to react to it as sugar, thus stimulating sugar cravings.

11. If the carbohydrate cravings are happening at night it may because this is the first time you are actually tuning in to your body. You also may need to track if you are eating enough earlier in the day or if you are eating enough protein and healthy fat at each meal.

12. Is there a healthy substitute for the desired food, equivalent in taste or texture? This may work for some of your cravings. *(See Appendix C for craving substitutions.)*

How to Eat a Highly Desired, "Trigger" Food

1. Mindfully: If you are going to eat, give yourself permission to really enjoy the food. Sit down at a table. Take food from the package/container and put it on a small plate, bowl or napkin. Focus on the food. No TV, computer, book or phone. Breathe–slow and relaxed. Take a bite, slowly chew the food, and really taste it. Take your time to engage all of your senses. Really taste it. Notice the color, flavor, texture, temperature, and aroma. Enjoy! This should help increase your feelings of satisfaction.

2. If it is sugar or a refined carbohydrate, try to eat it with protein or fiber, with a meal, or at the end of a meal. This will help balance your blood sugar, decrease rebound cravings, and help you be satisfied with a smaller amount.

3. Some individuals need to eat the trigger food with someone present and some individuals prefer to keep the high-risk food out of the house and eat it at a restaurant.

4. There may be a food you choose to avoid because it triggers an over-eating episode. Habituation (repeated planned exposure to the food using the above guidelines) is a helpful strategy. When you know you can actually have the forbidden food again, you will be less likely to overeat, and you will be more likely to eat a smaller portion or order a smaller size when you are using the planning and compensating strategies.

Give Yourself Permission to Emotionally Eat

- The reality is – you do have a choice of whether or not you use food to deal with issues, but you need to change the paradigm. Instead of being impulsive, compulsive, or zoned-out – be intentional. Be mindful.

- This prescription is less risky once you have developed a "grab bag" full of healthy alternatives to eating emotionally **and** if on most occasions, you are choosing those alternatives versus using food.

- Utilize your Awareness Record, Recipe Cards, and Bridge Flow Chart (Appendix D, E, F).

- As part of *Eating with Awareness*, when you have the urge to eat, if you have identified an emotional trigger, remember, you always have 3 choices:

  1. Use a healthy coping mechanism instead.
  2. If you don't want to, or aren't ready to deal with the issue, use a healthy avoidance strategy.
  3. You get to decide if you want to use food at this time. *(Be aware of the "ghost" – see Diet Mentality chapter.)*

- If you decide to eat to "self-medicate,"

  1. Eat mindfully (See How to Eat Highly Desired Food.)
  2. Find the right "small dose" of the "food of choice" that is just enough to comfort you without the side-effects you don't want.

- You may discover, the amount of food that is required to alter your emotional state is less than you think.

Chapter 1 Recap

√ Change in mindset from a "diet" focus to a health focus.

√ Eat with awareness – of how food makes your body feel.

√ Increase whole foods and water intake.

√ Increase fiber, non-starchy vegetables, healthy fat, lean or plant protein.

√ Decrease sugar, refined carbohydrates, and processed foods.

√ Eat mindfully.

√ Focus on internal cues for hunger and satiety.

√ Use Balance strategies: Tier approach and "planning and compensating".

√ Revisit your goals and "big why" every day (to help maintain motivation).

Chapter 2 Summary

- Are You an Emotional Eater?
- The Role of Food
- Family-of-origin and other Childhood Issues
- Trauma and Disordered Eating
- Unresolved Grief and Loss
- Stress
- Finding Value in Your Inner Beauty
- Your Mask and Shadow
- Personality Type and Eating Behavior
- Filling the Void: Relationships, Spirituality
- Awareness Record
- Creating a Bridge Between Mood and Food
- "Recipe Cards" for Alternative Behaviors
- Stress Management Strategies
- Physical Activity/Movement
- Restorative Practices

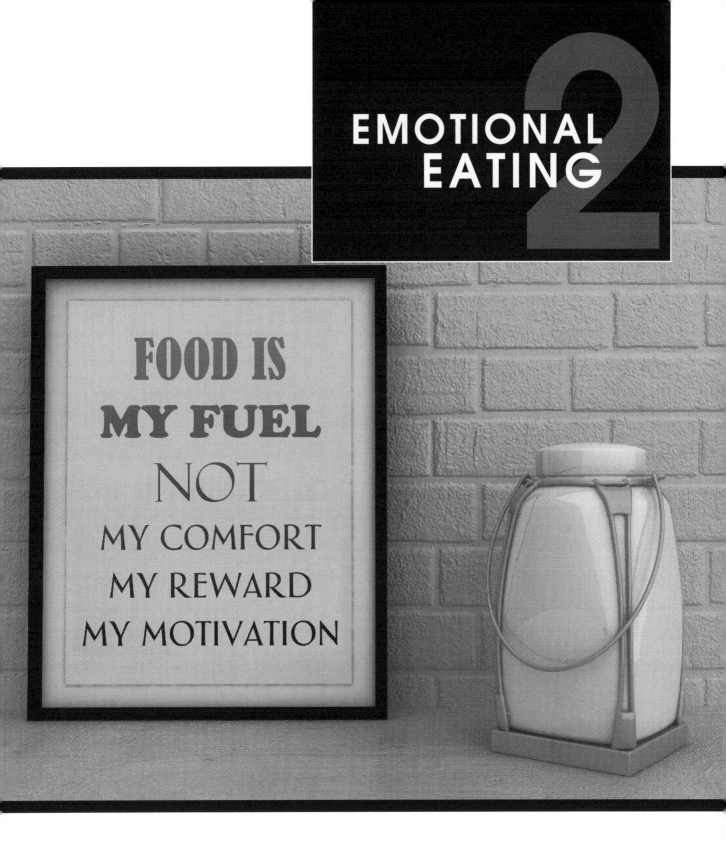

FOOD IS
MY FUEL
NOT
MY COMFORT
MY REWARD
MY MOTIVATION

"If you really want to make a friend, go to someone's house and eat with him . . . The people who give you their food give you their heart." – Cesar Chavez

Does food control your life? Are you tired of obsessing about food all day? Are you done letting what you eat and what the scale says determine your mood or how you feel about yourself? Even if you don't have an actual eating disorder, chronic dieting and constant body-image dissatisfaction can wear away at your health, happiness, and self-esteem.

You can heal emotional eating and change the role that food plays in your life. The glow approach will guide you in making peace with yourself, your body, and your relationship with food.

Emotional/Compulsive Eating is the Symptom — Not the Problem.

The real issue of disordered eating is not food, although food, eating and body image have enormous symbolic value. Worrying about food and weight may be a smokescreen to avoid dealing with other issues, as dieting is a culturally channeled outlet (Root, 1987). Obsessing about food and weight is a way to defocus off other issues. Recovery means discovering the purpose of the symptom. Compulsive eating is the symptom, not the problem. But in order to let it go, there needs to be something to fill the void or take its place.

Emotional Hunger is Symbolic — for Your "Inner Voice"

Hunger may be symbolic and represent a number of other unsatisfied needs. As you explore other issues, you will gain more awareness of the purpose the symptoms might serve. Increasing awareness means listening to your "hunger" – your inner voice (Chernin, 1986; Orbach, 1979; Roth, 1983). When you have an urge to eat, you will learn to differentiate between physical and psychological (emotional) hunger. You need to be willing to start feeling your emotions.

Stop. Breathe. Reflect. What are you feeling? What do you need? What are you trying to avoid or numb out? What do you expect this food to do for you? What else might your body need – water... rest... physical release... connection?

The *glow approach* will help you explore underlying issues that may be connected to the emotional eating and also rule out whether or not there is an actual disordered eating pattern present.

Are You an Emotional Eater?

- Do you turn to food when you are angry, anxious, sad, lonely, stressed, bored or need a "lift" in mood?

- Do you have difficulty tolerating strong emotions?

- Do you use food to self-soothe, numb-out, avoid, or procrastinate?
- Do you eat when you're not hungry?
- Do you tend to be passive and "stuff" your feelings or avoid conflict?
- Do you feel empty, void, or lack in other areas of your life?
- Do you feel you are deficient in coping skills?

If you answered yes to any of these questions, you may be using food to alter your emotional state. Emotional eating becomes problematic when the behavior becomes a pattern that you feel like you have no control over or it causes problems in your daily life (i.e., feelings of shame or guilt, low self-esteem, relationship issues and/or social avoidance, financial loss, or health problems because of poor nutrition or weight). Emotional eating may be a part of a symptom cluster that makes up disordered eating including bulimia, binge- eating disorder, anorexia, or orthorexia.

As you continue to use this workbook, my hope is that you are able to gain deeper awareness into your emotional eating patterns, and that you are able to develop other alternatives to manage those feelings, meet your needs, and find hope and healing on this journey of transformation.

The Role of Food

Food holds enormous symbolism in our culture. Food is pleasurable, and it is associated with nurturance and celebrations (social connection), reward and punishment, social status, control, etc. Food is not your enemy, nor is it meant to be your friend. For many people, food has become a substance used to alter mood.

We need to move food out of these roles and put it back into its primary role of providing nourishment for our body. "Eating with awareness" includes being aware of how you are feeling emotionally when you have the urge to eat so you can learn to differentiate between physical (when you need food) and emotional hunger (when you need something else). You need to be willing to feel and allow your emotions to surface. Emotional eating stuffs feelings, quiets your voice, and detaches you from your authentic self.

Emotional Hunger and Emotional Regulation

Emotional regulation is the ability to cope with emotions in a healthy way without using dysfunctional behavior. Emotional hunger is created when you don't have the ability to distinguish other emotions from physical hunger. Thus, eating is used to regulate those emotions.

You might be thinking, "I'm not sure if I even know what emotion I am feeling, let alone distinguishing an emotional state from being hungry." You are not alone. Many individuals with disordered eating feel out of touch with what they are feeling. I will discuss how this pattern often has its origin in childhood in the section on family-of origin.

We feel many of our emotions in our body's core, as emotions have a physiological component to them. Stress, worry, or anger can feel like nausea or butterflies in our stomach. Sadness, loss, or grief can feel like emptiness in the pit of our stomach or an ache in our heart. Since we associate physical hunger with sensations in our abdomen (located in our core), it is understandable that we may have difficulty differentiating between emotional and physical hunger.

As a child, you may not have known how to deal with those negative emotions. There may have been a lack of role modeling with using healthy coping skills. If it was an addictive environment, substances were being used to deal with life. Food is available and pleasurable, so a pattern of self-soothing with food begins. Once you cross that threshold, your mind/body remembers the association between that emotion and "feeling better" from eating.

The pattern that began in childhood can continue into adulthood and generalize to other emotions. If you have difficulty identifying feelings and you misinterpret emotions as hunger, the state is set for emotional eating. When you misread internal signals (feelings = hunger) you stop connecting with your authentic self.

There are two constructs that are often mentioned in the literature on mental health/eating disorders: alexithymia and interoceptive awareness (Cochrane et al, 1993; Herbert et al, 2013; Sokol et al).

Alexithymia is defined as a constriction of emotional functioning, an inability to identify and express or describe one's feelings, and difficulty distinguishing between emotions and bodily sensations. Individuals with high levels of alexithymia are usually aware of their emotional arousal, however, they have difficulty differentiating emotions and verbalizing them. Cochrane et al (1993) describes the adaptive function of eating disorder symptoms as related to alexithymia.

Interoceptive awareness is a sensitivity to stimuli origination in the body and an ability to perceive and identify internal signals. Individuals who have eating disorders typically have low interoceptive awareness as compared to individuals who are psychosomatic or hypochondriacal who have high interoceptive awareness. Interoseptive awareness includes appetite awareness and emotional awareness.

Low awareness of hunger and satiety cues as well as low emotional awareness may play an important role in emotional eating (Sokol et al). Do you identify with any of the above constructs?

_____

_____

_____

Many emotional eaters have difficulty with emotional regulation, as do individuals who struggle with other addictions and mental health conditions, including anxiety disorders, ADHD, bipolar disorder, PTSD, and BPD. Emotional regulation includes a number of skills:

1. Identify and Label
   - Differentiation (distinguish one type of emotion from another).
   - Modulate (identify level or intensity of emotion).
   - Integrate (able to blend different emotional states, i.e., love/hate).

2) Tolerate
   - Use emotion as a signal, not a trigger to act impulsively or numb-out.
   √ Use mindfulness and distress tolerance strategies.

3) Desomatization
   - Transition from experiencing emotions just on a physical level to using words to label how you are feeling. This will help you externalize your emotional experience and guide you to the next step.

4) Choose Coping Response
   - There are a variety of coping mechanisms available to assist you in identifying and managing your feelings. I will include many of these strategies at the end of this chapter and in the Appendix section, including _glow_'s "Awareness record," the "Bridge between food and mood" flowchart, and "recipe cards" for alternative behaviors to use instead of emotional eating.

Food Works! In the moment, comfort foods (high sugar and fat content) are pleasurable, thus distracting from the unpleasant emotion you are experiencing. Carbohydrates and fat trigger the release of your "feel good" chemicals (serotonin and endorphins) that evoke a state of calm and increased well-being. Even anticipating eating these foods will trigger your dopamine (reward system) which lifts your mood (see Physiology chapter). Eating/overeating/bingeing gives you something concrete to do so your focus is on food and not on the issue. Food works on an emotional, physiological, and behavioral level. It is your body's solution to a problem.

So, isn't it time for **no more guilt or shame?!** Guilt means you have done something wrong; shame means there is something wrong with you. Neither is correct. As a child, you found a way to self-soothe when you had no other skills available and/or no role-model to demonstrate healthy alternatives.

Even though food works, it is only temporary and the original problem remains. There also may be consequences from unhealthy food choices, overeating, or the added weight gain. You are in charge of your life. You now have a choice to learn new patterns and begin your journey of transformation. You are not alone.

This chapter is divided into subchapters that have some type of connection to emotional eating. You may choose to skip over the parts that don't pertain to you or jump ahead to the strategy section. This is your journey, your plan.

Family of Origin and Other Childhood Issues

Family-of-Origin

One of the primary functions of the family unit is to provide children with a safe and secure environment where they can achieve mastery over many different challenges. The family is where you are taught basic beliefs and values. In a healthy family, the rules are open for discussion and are often flexible. Children have the right to express thoughts and feelings, even when other family members don't agree and they are still accepted for their differences. Communication is open, direct, and respectful. No one person has all of the power. There is unconditional love. Children learn who they are and what to expect from life and begin to develop their sense of identity. If you were raised in a healthy family environment where you were valued, loved, and nurtured, then chances are you learned to feel good about yourself because you were shown that others felt good about you.

If you grew up in a dysfunctional family, the problems in your home could have been exhibited in many ways, including: alcohol or drug addiction, eating disorders, gambling, workaholism, or other addictive behavior; as well as mental health issues; chronic medical conditions by a parent or sibling; verbal, physical, or sexual abuse; neglect, including a narcissistic parent or any other disruption of healthy family interaction that results in a non-nurturing environment.

Separation, divorce, or inconsistent guardianship (including foster care or a parent who is incarcerated), may impact a child emotionally. The death of a parent or sibling may also have negative influences on a child's development.

When dysfunction exists in a home, the focus is usually on the dysfunctional parent or parents. The needs of the children are neglected, so they come to believe their needs don't matter. Without the encouragement, support, and love of a nurturing environment, you may have grown up thinking that you have no value. You may have not been given praise or affirmation. Instead, you may have heard criticism, mixed messages, or cool indifference. You may have learned to not feel good about yourself because others didn't treat you as if you were valued.

You may have learned to suppress your feelings, because no one responded, reactions were unpredictable, or you were silenced by someone's rage. It may not have been safe to communicate openly or directly. You may have learned to keep your thoughts to yourself, because you would have been rejected or told you were "talking back."

Conflicts may have been handled poorly. There may have been conflict avoidant behavior where problems were minimized or denied. There may have been passive-aggressive behavior displayed by the "cold shoulder," pay-backs, or conditional acceptance. There may have been over-reactivity or out-of-control anger and aggression displayed. Your family may have operated from crisis to crisis.

There may have been poor boundaries on multiple levels (role-reversals, privacy, etc.). There may have been inconsistent rules that you weren't allowed to question. If your parent was a perfectionist, narcissistic, or had OCD, you may have internalized negative messages that were told to you directly or were communicated indirectly by the way your parent treated you.

When you grow up in a dysfunctional home, rarely are you shown what real love really is. Often love is shown in negative or abusive ways. Because you grow up with negative feelings of what love is, you may have difficulty loving yourself or feeling that you deserve to be loved. If you grow up with a lack of nurturance, then you may not have learned how to nurture yourself.

Carolyn Coker Ross, MD, MPH addresses the issue of insecure attachment styles and their impact on disordered eating in *The Emotional Eating Workbook*. Your parent's response to you when you were distressed plays a role in how you connect with other people and how you respond to your own needs. Poor attachment with caretakers leads to poor nurturing of self. You may be able to ignore body cues for hunger or fullness, or your emotions may feel overwhelming and you may use food to numb-out. Food/eating can be a predictable experience if people are not.

Other types of dysfunctional family environments may include enmeshment – where there is intense over-involvement, lack of privacy, and autonomy is seen as disloyal; the overprotective environment – where separation- individuation is blunted, and decision making is governed by the parent; the perfectionistic environment where achievement is highly valued, and there is an emphasis on appearance, status, and family reputation. This environment may also prohibit negative feelings, minimize personal problems, and use conditional approval. Parents may come across as critical and judgmental, and the child may not ever feel good enough.

ACOA (Adult Children of an Alcoholic)

Growing up in a home where there are addictions can be unpredictable. There are many different characteristics that are commonly seen in an ACOA (Woititz, 1983). These characteristics also depend on the role the child was ascribed or took on.

If the parent isn't emotionally available, the child often becomes parentified. This characteristic encompasses taking on or being given a role or duties that are beyond the child's emotional maturity in order to meet the needs of the adult. The child hopes to attain acceptance and approval. A caretaking pattern often develops from this role, having been conditioned to anticipate the needs and feelings of others in an attempt to gain control in a chaotic environment.

If the parent in an addictive environment uses substances to manage emotions, this role-modeling may set the stage for a child to use food as a substance to self-regulate, especially if people aren't safe or available.

If there is no one there to comfort, affirm, or tell you that it is going to be okay – and that you are okay, then there are no positive messages to internalize. Internalized messages create the foundation for our own self-talk. If there are no internal resources and no external support then substances provide the external means to comfort, sooth, distract, release, contain, avoid, and numb-out (Root, Fallon, and Friedrich, 1986).

Re-Enactments (Recreating the Past, in the Present)

The patterns that might develop from growing up in a dysfunctional family include:

- Suppressing thoughts and feelings that might bring on rejection
- Difficulty with emotional regulation
- Poor communication skills
- Difficulty with assertiveness and boundaries
- Conflict avoidant
- Suppressing own needs
- Need for approval
- People-pleasing
- Caretaking
- Perfectionism
- Learned helplessness
- Issues with control
- Low self-esteem and lack of identity
- Issues with trust and relationship difficulties
- Lack of self-nurturing and coping skills

We will address how these patterns may play out in food and weight issues and in the "purpose of the symptoms."

You may not identify with any of the above patterns. Sometimes the association between food and other emotions is subtle. In every culture, sharing a meal is a sign of acceptance, inclusion, and caring. Visualize a mother feeding her baby – the ultimate bonding experience. You may have been raised to associate food with love, security, and celebration. There may have been food insecurity because of poverty. Perhaps your parents lived through the Great Depression or another food shortage experience.

You may have grown up in an appearance focused environment, been involved in a sport or activity that was weight or body shape focused, or you may have gotten comments from a boyfriend/girlfriend or coach. There may have been disordered eating patterns demonstrated in your home, including chronic dieting, emotional eating, or another type of eating disorder. As an adult, you may be repeating the eating patterns you had as a child, from fast food or junk food to traditional farm-style eating (not a match with today's more sedentary lifestyle).

As you pause and reflect on what you have read, what are your thoughts or feelings?

_____

_____

_____

_____

_____

_____

The Relationship between Trauma and Eating Disorders

The research has long established that trauma histories are associated with eating disorders, especially among binge eating or purging type (Brewerton, 2007; Gay, 1997; Pershing, 2014). The spectrum of trauma experiences includes not only childhood sexual abuse, but date/acquaintance rape, physical abuse and assault, emotional abuse, and emotional and physical neglect (including food deprivation or scarcity), sexual harassment, sexual assault during adulthood, domestic violence, teasing, and bullying. Any experience that can produce PTSD may increase the probability of developing disordered eating (Talbot et al., 2013). Trauma-related disorders include mood and anxiety disorders, eating disorders and substance abuse, dissociative, somatoform, impulse control and disruptive disorders, and several of the personality disorders, including BPD, as well as a variety of medical conditions.

Trauma has a powerful impact on the brain and body, including the central and autonomic nervous system. Trauma triggers the fight, flight, or freeze response. This causes a surge of adrenalin and cortisol which can then set forth a series of bodily dysregulation, especially if the stress is chronic (Van der Kolk, 1994).

The" toxic stress" response, (as coined by Jack P. Shonkoff, Director of the Center for the Developing Child at Harvard University) can occur when a child experiences strong, frequent, and/or prolonged adversity such as physical, sexual, or emotional abuse, chronic neglect, caregiver substance abuse or mental illness, exposure to violence, and/or the accumulated burdens of family economic hardship – especially in the absence of supportive caregiving from adults.

Chronic stress creates elevated levels of cortisol, which can damage the hippocampus, leading to depression and memory problems. A decrease in hippocampus size is associated with greater risk of dissociative symptoms (Bowers, 2005). This coping mechanism of dissociation learned during trauma can become automatic and generalize to other situations of distress. High cortisol levels also trigger hunger. Eating/overeating/bingeing can become the gateway to re-enact dissociation (numbing-out or avoidance) of present day stressors (Iazetto, 1989).

The "kindling effect" has been used to describe the neurological tendency of the brain to become over-sensitized following exposure to trauma (Van der Kolk et al, 1995). The result is the lowering of an individual's threshold to trauma, making the individual both more susceptible to re-traumatization as well as re-victimization. This is often experienced present day as over-reactivity and hypersensitivity to possible threat, and for an emotional eater, food has become the coping mechanism to manage this constant feeling of stress.

Sexual Abuse and Disordered Eating

It has been clearly established in the research that childhood sexual abuse is a significant risk factor for eating disorders, (Gregory-Bills, 1990; Schwartz and Gay, 1996; Shroyer-Small, 1992; Small and Jackson, 1989; Wooley and Kearney-Cooke, 1986), including BED (Pershing, 2014) and other psychiatric disorders. The utilization of an eating disorder as a coping response can be seen as a regressive developmental retreat. Erikson (1968) suggests that developmental damage can occur when a child is traumatized beyond their ability to cope. A child's development is arrested at the age at which the abuse begins; identity, autonomy, object relations, and body-image can be impacted. If trauma occurs at a stage when the child is functioning concretely, then she may not learn to express herself verbally or cope abstractly (cognitive problem solving). Romeo (1984) suggests that non-verbal behaviors, i.e. body language, become a source of communication when the ego is overwhelmed with anxiety. An eating disorder may be a method of coping for women who have not developed healthy skills for coping with the negative feelings, images, or thoughts accompanying sexual trauma (Root, 1989). Disordered eating can be used to displace thoughts and feelings about the abuse onto the culturally sanctioned preoccupation with food and weight. Compulsive behavior may leave little time to think about anything else.

Original defenses used at the time of the abuse form the survivor's later core coping responses, i.e., dissociation, splitting (good/bad), personalization (self-blame). Thus, when a survivor is experiencing present day stress, she may regress and utilize eating disorder symptoms to dissociate or defocus on concrete issues such as food, weight, and body-image.

Due to the high level of egocentricity in childhood and thus a tendency for self-blame, the survivor will often see herself as bad and will self-punish by restricting or bingeing (over-eating to the point of pain). Overeating creates strong bodily sensations that help defocus or distract from emotions. Memories of the trauma may be replaced with less distressing preoccupation with food. Now food is good or bad, and self is good or bad depending on which food is eaten. Unresolved guilt and shame about the abuse gets projected onto eating behavior and body-image: "The abuse was bad, I'm bad, my body's bad, my body is fat. I can fix it by losing weight." (Body-image and the scale are concrete images.) The body becomes the battle ground for acting out repressed feelings (Wooley and Wooley, 1986). She disrespects her body so she does not nourish it properly.

The need for control that is seen in survivors with disordered eating relates to the feelings of helplessness during the abuse. Feelings of powerlessness are displaced onto the body by defocusing on feeling out of control with bingeing. This pattern of learned helplessness can carry over into present day, as most chronic dieters express the feeling that they are not able to have control over their eating, or that they feel hopeless and helpless about sticking to a "diet." Regaining a sense of control may mean starting a new "diet" with rules to follow and promoting a sense of restraint. The survivor did not have control over her body during the abuse, so now she uses food, weight, and her body to maintain a sense of control (Root and Fallon, 1988).

An exaggerated preoccupation with the body, powerlessness, and need for control may be present in the survivor (Meiselman, 1990). When a child lacks a sense of personal power and worth, she may base her feelings of self-esteem on losing weight and achieving a socially valued ideal (thin) body (Bruch, 1973). Sexual abuse exaggerates the significance of the body in defining self. Self- identity may be expressed via an over valuing of body-image as representative of self.

The abuse survivor experiences low self-esteem as a result of the abuse; losing weight and having the "ideal" body has cultural value. She feels that if she is perfect (thin), no one will notice that she has been abused (damaged). She feels different because of the abuse; having food/weight issues helps her to defocus and feel different because of being overweight or having disordered eating (Kearney-Cooke, 1988).

An eating disorder may be used as an attempt to set boundaries and create personal space (O'brien, 1987). Gaining weight may be an unconscious attempt to avoid being noticed; extra weight may be used as protection. Weight loss invites unwanted attention; she may feel objectified, which may trigger memories of the abuse. Eating and weight may be used as a way to avoid sexual intimacy or turn off sexual feelings. If there is a fear to get close to people in general, she may use weight as an excuse to not socialize.

There are multiple themes that emerge when one begins to look at the connection between sexual abuse and disordered eating. The most visible theme is related to body-image and the symbolism that is played out in the disordered eating and weight patterns (Root, 1987; Wooley and Kearney-Cooke, 1987).

Beginning Your Healing Journey

As you take time to process what you have just read, it is often helpful to write out your thoughts and feelings. You may have gained some insights into your own background and impact on your food/weight history. Depending on your story, it may be helpful to seek professional help to guide you in your recovery process.

You may have kept the lid on "Pandora's box" for a long time, using a variety of coping mechanisms that suppress feelings or memories (eating, substance use, dissociation), but you may also have felt its toll with depression, anxiety, and rage. It is not unusual to see an escalation in symptoms when you start purposefully remembering.

Thus, in order to take a look at your past, it is important to be prepared psychologically with new, healthy coping mechanisms in order to tolerate the emotions that arise with processing traumatic memories. Prep work includes being taught or already knowing "grounding techniques," "safe place" imagery, relaxation strategies, and cognitive restructuring.

Since most of "past" work is actually grief work, it is important that you include someone that you trust to walk this healing journey with you. If you are not yet seeing a counselor who works with trauma, and you start experiencing overwhelming symptoms (depression, anxiety, insomnia, suicidal or self-harm thoughts, etc.) – please seek help immediately.

Thoughts, feelings, or insights: _____

_____

_____

_____

_____

_____

Unresolved Grief and Loss

The impact of an early loss of a parental figure can stay with a child long into adulthood. Comfort foods that were associated with nurturing from this person may be used in the present to "symbolically" reconnect.

Loss can occur at any age in an individual's life and still be traumatic. You may be well aware of the loss of a significant other in your life – a child, spouse, parent, sibling, or other close relation or friend. Grief not only occurs after a death, but other losses as well.

When you review your loss history, does it include any of the following?

☐ Divorce, separation ☐ Loss of a pet

☐ Difficult break-up with dating partner ☐ Miscarriage(s)

☐ Loss of job, retirement ☐ Infertility

☐ Loss of health ☐ Abortion

☐ Loss of a significant friendship ☐ Giving a child up for adoption

☐ Son or daughter leaving home ☐ Being adopted

☐ Multiple moves (neighborhood, city, state, country) ☐ Loss of dignity/reputation/self-respect

☐ Loss of home (natural disaster, fire, financial) ☐ Traumatic death (suicide, murder, military)

☐ Other

It is often helpful to diagram a chronological loss history by year and age, and add any other relevant information (when emotional eating began, weight history, etc.). Narrative journaling is helpful with exploring your feelings about the loss, the effects the loss had on your life, and whether or not it is still impacting you. (You may want to use a separate journal for this exercise.)

Chronological Loss History

Example:

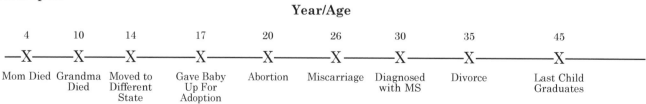

Year/Age

4	10	14	17	20	26	30	35	45
—X—	—X—	—X—	—X—	—X—	—X—	—X—	—X—	—X—
Mom Died	Grandma Died	Moved to Different State	Gave Baby Up For Adoption	Abortion	Miscarriage	Diagnosed with MS	Divorce	Last Child Graduates

Type of Loss (x)

Your Loss History

Year/Age

_____

Type of Loss (x)

Thoughts or feelings after processing the above exercise _____

_____

_____

_____

_____

_____

_____

_____

_____

_____

Loss is often felt as "emptiness" or a "void". Food can be used to fill that void and as a means to "self-medicate." Emotional eating can be a way to self-soothe, distract, or avoid "feeling the feelings." Grief work is a combination of dealing with the loss (strategies), healthy distraction, and having a support network. This may involve:

√ Grief counseling and/or grief support group.

√ Getting support from family and friends.

√ Expressive therapies: journaling, art, music, etc.

√ Spirituality.

√ "Recipe cards" for self-soothing and healthy avoidance.

Current Stressors

Is there anything going on in your life that is causing you stress?

- ☐ Relationship difficulties
- ☐ Being harassed, bullied, or abused
- ☐ Parenting
- ☐ Pregnancy
- ☐ Job or school issues
- ☐ Retirement

- ☐ Financial
- ☐ Legal
- ☐ Health
- ☐ Spiritual
- ☐ Sexual
- ☐ Home environment or change in living conditions

☐ Other _____

How are you coping with it? _____

_____

_____

Are you using food to avoid, distract, or self-soothe? _____

_____

_____

What can you do instead? _____

_____

_____

Self-Esteem/Self-Identity: Finding Value in your Inner Beauty

Self-esteem is a sense of your own worth, your self-evaluation of who you are (self-identity). Your self-identity is a collection of beliefs about how you see yourself including your personality attributes, character, values, skills and abilities, intellect, occupation, hobbies, spirituality, gender, race, sexual orientation, and physical attributes. Our self-esteem and self-identity influences our behaviors, perceptions, mood, and many of our life choices including friendships, mates, and occupation.

Our self-development is largely influenced by our early social interactions and the feedback we get from others (introjections) until we are old enough and have the cognitive abilities to interpret our own feelings and abilities. (Watkins, 1978) discuss the concept of ego states: significant others (caretakers) help label the child's emotional states and let the child know that the emotion/behavior is ok. If the emotion is not validated, the child makes a split and compartmentalizes what others can't tolerate (anger, individuality, sexuality, independence, etc.). Children need a sense that they are loved and approved of, so they become what they think others want them to be (compliant, perfect, achievement oriented, etc.). This is known as the "false self."

(Torem, 1987) and (Gay, 1997), utilize these constructs in reframing eating disordered (ED) symptoms as serving a purpose with helping to maintain the false self. Once you identify what aspect of the self the ED behavior is trying to manage you can then replace old patterns with a new pattern of behavior that is age-appropriate, satisfies the original intent, and is not a re-enactment from the past.

As you discover your true self, you will begin to secure a more solid self-identity. When you begin to explore, understand, and own all parts of yourself, you will experience an increase in your self-esteem. Are you familiar with the self-statement, "If people really knew me, they wouldn't like me"? You may be describing your false self (the masks you wear that you know will bring approval, and your shadow – the parts you hide that you fear will bring rejection). Healing begins when you "deconstruct" the masks you wear and when you "make friends" with your shadow side. Once you let go of these "compensatory" strategies, your true "authentic" self will emerge.

Exploring Your False-Self

Mask "I need to be this way for people to like or accept me."

> *Examples: thin, happy, perfect, caretaker, people-pleaser, passive, good, successful, sexy, etc.*

Your Mask:

_____

_____

_____

Shadow "Parts of me that aren't okay and will bring rejection."

Examples: anger, weakness, sadness, sexuality issues, diversity, etc.

Your Shadow Side:

_____

_____

_____

Deconstructing the Mask

Don't worry; you will not become an empty shell if you decide to let go of your false self. I will get you started on how the process works. If we put each of the characteristics on a spectrum, there is probably an aspect of it that really is who you are, and not only is it not harmful; it is actually okay. It becomes problematic when you take it to an extreme or feel that it is a role you have to take on in order to be liked or accepted. It is a problem if you ignore your inner voice that is feeling resentment/tired/unsure; it is letting you know that you have a boundary that may have been crossed.

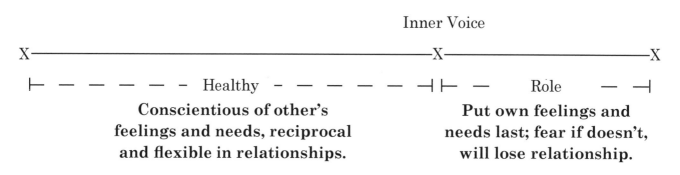

Inner Voice

X————————————————————X————————————————X

├ — — — — — – Healthy - — — — — — ┤├ — Role — ┤

Conscientious of other's feelings and needs, reciprocal and flexible in relationships.   **Put own feelings and needs last; fear if doesn't, will lose relationship.**

Example: People-Pleaser

Explore: *Ava grew up in a home with a mother who was critical and a father who over-reacted to everything. Ava was constantly "walking on eggshells," trying to not upset her father and gain the approval of her mother. She became very good at becoming what would keep the peace in her family. Trying to make others happy became the means to maintain control over how they might react to her. Ava continues this pattern in her adult life, especially in her dating relationships. She often ends up with men who are self-centered and don't reciprocate.*

How ED Symptom May Maintain this Role:

If you are constantly putting your own needs last, you may be using food as self-nurturance or to suppress (stuff) your true feelings. People-pleasing can also create a lot of anxiety by always worrying about making other people happy. Eating can become a way to manage this anxiety and change your focus from what you may think you are doing wrong.

Alternative Coping Strategy:

A new pattern could be – continue to be your gracious self, but also honor your feelings and needs. Healthy relationships will support the changes you are making. Taking off the mask means that Ava can continue to be her natural amiable, flexible, helpful self, but it also helps her to not lose her sense of self in a relationship. She can be honest about how she is feeling, and can say no or set limits. People-pleasing also benefits from cognitive restructuring strategies and self-identity enhancing skills.

Example: Caretaking

Explore: *Elizabeth grew up in a home where she was the oldest of 6 children. Both of her parents worked to make ends meet. She did most of the cooking and took care of her younger siblings. Her mother became ill with Multiple Sclerosis and Elizabeth took on most of her care-giving as well. Elizabeth continued this socially endorsed pattern when she married her high-school sweetheart, who had problems with drug and alcohol abuse. Unsurprisingly, she is employed as a nurse at the local hospital.*

How ED Symptoms May Maintain this Role:

After working all day, Elizabeth comes home and gets dinner started. She puts a load of laundry in while her husband sits in front of the TV drinking a beer. After dinner, she cleans up the kitchen and he falls asleep on the couch. She bathes the children, gets them ready for bed, and then collapses in front of the TV with a bowl of ice-cream. Eating is how she nurtures herself, fills the void of intimacy that is lacking with her husband, and defocuses off of her marital issues.

Alternative Coping Strategy:

Elizabeth has some family-of-origin work to do to help her disengage from the re-enactment she is in with this role. She needs to give herself permission to nurture herself in other ways besides food – a warm bath, a massage, painting her nails, prayer, reaching out to family and friends, or setting limits with her husband. (She may need the support of a marital counselor.) Elizabeth can continue to be the caring mother, nurse, friend, and wife that she always was, while getting her needs met as well and not always doing for others – especially another adult – what they should be doing for themselves.

Continue this exercise with each of your Masks and identify how ED symptoms may be serving a purpose or helping maintain that role. In order to give up a symptom, you need to replace it with an alternative, something that meets the original intent.

Mask _____

ED symptom/purpose_____

_____

_____

_____

Alternative coping strategy _____

_____

_____

_____

Mask _____

ED symptom/purpose_____

_____

_____

_____

Alternative coping strategy _____

_____

_____

"Making Friends" with Your Shadow

Yikes, does this sound scary? Probably because you are looking at those parts of you through the eyes of your "inner child" or as a critical introject (someone else's viewpoint that you internalized). We will use cognitive restructuring and compassionate insight to reframe how you view those behaviors, as most of them are actually symptoms.

Example: It's not okay to be angry.

Explore: Mary grew up in a home where anger was either not expressed or was shown as rage (screaming, swearing, or out of control behavior). Father was an abusive alcoholic and Mother was a compulsive eater and overweight.

How ED Symptom May Maintain this Behavior:

When Mary feels angry with someone, she can feel her body reacting – heart rate and breathing increases, muscles tense– but she doesn't want to get angry, i.e., lose control. This is often a trigger for a binge or over-eating episode. The food calms her and gives her something to focus on.

Compassionate Insight and Other Alternative Coping Strategies:

Mary associates anger with her father's rage episodes. Mary needs to differentiate anger from rage. Anger as an emotion is okay; it's a signal to let us know that we need to check in with our experience. Assertiveness training can help with teaching healthy ways to express anger while respecting others and ourselves.

Example: "Promiscuity"

Explore: Karen felt a lot of shame about how many sexual partners she had in the past. She was overweight and had not dated in years. She lost the same 20 pounds over and over again. Karen shares that, as a child, she was molested, and as a teen, she had difficulty saying no to sexual advances.

How ED Symptoms May Serve a Purpose:

Karen shared that when she loses weight, men start to notice her more often. This makes her feel very self-conscious, so she retreats to her home and the overeating begins again. The focus on the dieting cycle keeps her from thinking about her past. When she is dieting, she feels in control. The overeating helps her to numb-out and avoid thinking about the present incident that had triggered thoughts about her past sexual behavior. By re-labeling promiscuity as sexual disinhibition, the gender-biased derogatory term/behavior becomes a neutral symptom. Then, she can stop loathing herself and begin to look at gaining insight into the symptom, as well as begin to heal the issues from her past.

Compassionate Insight and Other Alternative Coping Strategies:

As we begin to explore Karen's childhood sexual abuse (CSA) history, we discuss some of the common sequela (aftereffects) of CSA, sexuality issues being one of the many. Sexual disinhibition can be an unconscious attempt to gain mastery/control or a type of learned helplessness (feeling like she doesn't have a choice and can't say no). She may have learned to overvalue the sexuality aspect of her identity and feels that it is the only way to be recognized. Gaining weight may be her way to establish a physical boundary to protect herself and keep others away, and also feel less sexualized.

Psychoeducation and counseling for her trauma and sequela is the first step of Karen's recovery. She will learn to have a voice, feel empowered, and be in charge of her sexual boundaries, no longer needing the extra weight to communicate for her.

Continue to explore the parts of you that you feel "aren't okay," and as you begin to integrate these aspects of yourself, you will no longer need the food/weight symptoms to cover up your shadow.

Shadow _____

How ED symptoms may maintain this behavior_____

_____

_____

_____

Compassionate insight and alternative coping strategies _____

_____

_____

Shadow _____

How ED symptom may serve a purpose:_____

_____

_____

_____

_____

Compassionate insight and alternative coping strategies:_____

_____

_____

_____

_____

Wrapping Things Up

Are there any more negative tapes running in your head about who you are: that you're not enough, that there is something wrong with you? Are you ready to let go of your old "life script"? Is that who you are today?

_____

_____

_____

_____

_____

_____

_____

_____

Personality Type (and impact on weight-loss success)

Personality is the combination of behavior, emotion, motivation, and thought patterns that define an individual. It's the way you view, understand and relate to the outside world, as well as how you see yourself. Personality forms during childhood, shaped through an interaction of your genes (temperament) and environment. There are close to 700 personality traits that have been defined and are categorized as positive, negative, or neutral. I have identified 10 that seem to play a role in impacting weight-loss including: perfectionist/compulsive, disorganized/procrastinator, caretaking/people-pleasing, dependent, self-critical/negative, impulsive, moody *(see Physiology chapter)*, rebellious/passive-aggressive, avoidant, and extrovert.

Perfectionist/Compulsive

- Do you see yourself as self-critical or have high expectations of yourself or others?
- Do you like to have a plan or have things done a certain way?
- Do you have an all/none thinking style?
- Do you have a high need for control?

The above characteristics may be simply traits or they may be part of a symptom cluster for another disorder, including anxiety disorders, obsessive- compulsive disorder, other addictions or eating disorders, or obsessive-compulsive personality disorder.

Strategies:

√ It's okay to look for a program that has a structured plan, but there also needs to be flexibility built in, such as using: Tier Approach, Planning/Compensating, and Plan B.

√ Reframe focus: Calorie counting may be a way to channel compulsiveness if there is an internal need to count or keep track (which may not be healthy for some individuals). An alternative can be tracking food groups, nutrients, or health.

√ Use Cognitive Restructuring: Challenge all/none thinking: (healthy choice/options vs. "right way," slip vs. relapse). *(See Diet Mentality chapter.)*

√ Try not to have too many "diet" rules to follow; be realistic and flexible. It doesn't need to be perfect – aim for balance.

√ Healthy distractions: Compulsive behaviors are often used as a way to avoid other issues. Develop a list for "healthy avoidance" alternatives until you feel ready to address the issues.

Disorganized/Procrastinator

- Explore why you think you have difficulty keeping things organized: too many things, too little space, too many people or responsibilities to keep track of, not enough time, or just overwhelmed? _____

  _____

  _____

- Explore why you think you procrastinate? Is the task unpleasant, boring, or overwhelming? Do you not know where or how to start? Do you feel it needs to be done perfectly so you don't start unless you can finish it a certain way? _____

  _____

  _____

- The above characteristics can be simply traits or they can be a part of a symptom cluster for ADD/ADHD, anxiety disorders, or OCD.

Strategies:

  √ Utilize a structured plan – with flexibility.

  √ Use of a daily planner: (shopping list, meal plan, and exercise schedule).

  √ Get it out of your head – write it down! (This will help increase motivation; decrease feelings of being overwhelmed; give you an opportunity to gain insight; and provide a venue for scheduling meal plans, exercise, relaxation, and other self-care.)

  √ Healthy avoidance strategies: If procrastination is a trigger to eat because what you need to do is unpleasant (food is pleasant and gives you something else to do), then you need to develop your list of healthy avoidance options. Now you have 3 options: i.e., if you need to complete an assignment and you don't feel like it that moment, instead of eating, you could read a book, go for a walk, etc. Always have back-up choices available.

  √ Utilize time-management strategies and prioritizing (to help with feelings of being overwhelmed).

  √ Build your skills for dealing with procrastination. Write down a task and then break it down into smaller, more manageable parts. Estimate how much time each part will take. Make a note of the actual time it took for future reference.

√ Mindful eating: When you're disorganized, you can also have difficulty with focusing, so you may not be focusing on satisfying "mouth hunger." Taking the time to sit down to eat and focus on your food can be centering.

Caretaking/People-Pleasing

- I have grouped these two styles together as they contain many similarities in their origin, role in self-identity/self-esteem, and difficulty with boundaries.

- Although family-of-origin plays a part in the development of personality and relational patterns, cultural influences infiltrate into our subconscious as well. The role of wife and mother (caregiver) was originally bestowed through biological gender differences. Femininity has been equated with being kind, nurturing, and self-sacrificing. Women have been socialized to be responsible for the needs of their family, nurturing everyone else but their needs may go unmet. The role of caretaker is culturally endorsed, and if vulnerable from FOO dynamics, a woman may take these patterns into adult relationships (i.e., ACOA melds into co-dependency). Codependency becomes role that provides self-esteem/identity, control, and a way to defocus off what needs to be taken care of in your own life by focusing on fixing someone else's.

Caretaking

- Does taking care of others (beyond what they really need) leave you little time to take care of yourself? Weight management does take time: meal planning, food preparation, packing lunches and snacks, exercise, etc. _____

_____

_____

- Ignoring your own needs – pretending that you don't matter – produces a pervasive sense of unfulfillment (void or emptiness). Are you using food to fill that void, nurture yourself, relax, self- sooth, or as a transition from work/family (i.e., crashing on the couch in front of the TV – chores done and everyone in bed – with a bag, bowl, or plate of food. Ahhhh… zone out time).

_____

_____

_____

Strategies:

√ Develop and implement self-care strategies: schedule time for taking care of you: relaxation/meditation, exercise/movement, rest, leisure, hobbies, social connection, spirituality, etc.

√ Set healthy limits and boundaries: It is okay to say no. Enabling others is not helping them or you. Learn to differentiate between caring for and taking care of. Address how the role is impacting you and your eating behavior.

√ Develop and insist upon reciprocal relationships. Your feelings and needs matter too. If you are feeling loved and cared for, it decreases the need for food to fill that void.

People-Pleasing

• Do you try to make others happy and gain their approval at the expense of your personal needs and feelings? _____

_____

_____

• Do you avoid expressing thoughts or feelings that may bring on disapproval, anger, or rejection? _____

_____

_____

• When you conform to someone else's expectations of you, you lose touch with your own feelings, needs, and beliefs (your inner self). This interferes with being able to develop a stable self-identity which fosters an internal locus of control. Thus, if unaware of self/needs, becomes preoccupied with others and depends on them for (external) approval/validation, which fosters insecurity and a wavering self-esteem. If your sense of self-worth depends on someone else's evaluation and approval, you will never be sure that you are okay.

Strategies:

√ Self-awareness strategies to help identify your own feelings and needs.

√ Self-identity and self-esteem building to guide looking within yourself for approval, direction, and validation.

√ Assertiveness training: maintaining healthy boundaries, setting limits, learning to say no.

Dependent

- Do you tend to be passive and submissive in your relationships? Do you feel inadequate in decision making or in taking care of yourself? _____

  _____

  _____

  _____

- Are you fearful of being alone? Do you feel that being in an unhealthy relationship is better than not being in a relationship? ((This personality type may be at risk for abusive relationships.) _____

  _____

  _____

  _____

- These traits may be a part of dependent personality disorder or co- occur with avoidant personality disorder or social anxiety, resulting in a limited support system.

Strategies:

√ Journaling and self-awareness record. (It may not be safe to verbalize feeling, yet you need an outlet to understand your inner feelings, fears, and needs and how those issues may be connected to your use of food.)

√ Assertiveness training – instead of "stuffing" feelings or using food/weight to indirectly communicate.

√ Self-esteem building to help you become aware of your inner strength and be able to have boundaries and set limits instead of using weight as an excuse to stay (i.e.., "No one else will want me if I look like this.").

√ Increase social support and/or spirituality.

√ Seek professional support if relationship is abusive. You need to develop a safety plan vs. using weight/size for safety.

(Caretaking, people pleasing, and dependent personality styles may be more at risk for abusive relationships or one where there is an addiction present.)

Self-Critical

Do you suffer from low self-esteem? Another way to describe this trait is lacking self-compassion or even self-verbal abuse. Do you have negative reactions to your mistakes?

- Defocusing on food/weight may take your focus off of the real issues. Example: If you are angry with yourself about how you handled a situation, you might look in the mirror and think, "I'm fat"; then the diet becomes the solution, versus looking at self or situation.

- If this is a daily pattern it may reflect core beliefs from unresolved childhood/family-of-origin issues or it may be a symptom of other disorders including: perfectionism, compulsiveness, OCD, OCPD, anxiety or depression, or borderline personality disorder.

Strategies:

√ Journaling and cognitive restructuring to challenge negative self-talk and assess for underlying core beliefs that also need to be healed.

√ Self-esteem work: including family of origin/childhood autobiography to assess what messages were internalized that are not healthy or true and begin to change 'life-script."

√ Learn to eat without shame – food is not a moral issue!

√ Self-forgiveness – Spirituality.

√ Set realistic goals.

√ Focus on behavior, not self. You are not your behavior. If you make a mistake or have a "slip," replace "I'm stupid, worthless, etc." with compassionate, non-judgmental self-talk (i.e., "It's okay, I'm human, everyone makes mistakes, what can I learn from this").

√ Body-image work.

Impulsive

- Do you have difficulty with restraint and/or do you speak or act before you think about

  the pros/cons or consequences? _____

  _____

  _____

  _____

  _____

- Do you focus on instant gratification versus long-term benefit? _____

_____

_____

_____

If impulsivity is a pattern for you, you may struggle with other addictions or other eating disorders and/or it may be a symptom of ADD/ADHD, BPD, or bipolar disorders.

Strategies:

√ Planning and structure: utilize a shopping list and have a meal plan; schedule your exercise in a day planner.

√ Use of environmental controls (awareness of food cues): Place healthful food in the front of cupboards or refrigerator. Place high-risk foods out of sight or do not bring them home (eat them at a restaurant or elsewhere so you can control the portion size). *(See Modify Your Environment.)*

√ Use of Journaling and Awareness Record to help organize your thoughts and slow down your response so you can utilize alternatives.

√ Schedule time for relaxation/meditation to help manage underlying physiology, *(see Physiology chapter).*

√ Have a plan for high-risk foods, *(see Nutrition or Sustainable Maintenance chapters).*

√ Mindful eating: Slow down and enjoy your food! *(See "mindful eating" exercise in Nutrition chapter.)*

Moody

- Are you prone to negative emotions, irritability, and/or do you see yourself as overly sensitive or emotionally reactive? _____

_____

_____

- Are you aware of self-medicating your mood with food?_____

_____

_____

- If you are moody more days than not, and it is a pattern for you, there may be an underlying mood disorder (depression, anxiety, bipolar, OCD, ADHD, PTSD, or borderline personality disorder).

- You may want to schedule an appointment with your physician to rule out a medical or hormonal condition (PMS, perimenopause, thyroid, etc. *(see Physiology chapter))*.

- Are there interpersonal issues that you may be suppressing? _____

_____

_____

_____

_____

Strategies:

√ Journal and Awareness Record: record symptoms/events/thoughts to see if there is a pattern and connection to emotional eating.

√ Cognitive restructuring to challenge negative thinking.

√ Self-soothing that doesn't involve food.

√ Exercise/relaxation – movement and meditation. *(See Physiology chapter.)*

√ Emotional regulation skills.

√ Restorative practice for emotional enhancement.

√ Assessment to rule out underlying co-morbidity and/ or treat underlying condition.

Rebellious/Passive-Aggressive

Rebellious

- Do you have a strong desire to resist authority, control, or convention?
- Do you describe yourself as a "free spirit"?
- Do others describe you as strong-willed or noncompliant?
- If this behavior has caused significant problems for you in relationships then there may be an underlying cause such as: ADHD, OCD, bipolar, BPD, or other personality disorders.

Passive-Aggressive

- When you rebel, do you do so openly and directly or is it more covert, i.e., passive-aggressive?
- Do you have difficulty with assertiveness or are you conflict-avoidant?

Strategies:

√ Choice: This is your plan! You create the rules, restrictions, or guidelines that you want to follow.

√ Start with small, simple, gradual changes.

√ Utilize Mindful Eating.

√ Be aware of the "ghost." Who is telling you that you can't eat? *(See Diet Mentality chapter.)*

√ Explore FOO: re-enactments and internalizations.

Avoidant

- Do you see yourself as shy or do you avoid personal relationships/social situations?

_____

_____

- If you avoid leaving your home, you may be exposed to multiple food cues. If you are lonely or bored, food may be main source of pleasure or fill the void. We associate comfort food with people. Comfort food reminds us of special moments and traditions – so we may turn to those foods to feel connected again.

- If you wish you had more relationships than you do or if fear is holding you back, then there may be an underlying condition such as social anxiety, agoraphobia, or other anxiety disorders.

Strategies:

√ Differentiate between social anxiety and introversion; one needs treatment and the other doesn't! Social anxiety is very treatable.

√ If you prefer to be home alone, *(see Modify Your Environment chapter)* to help decrease food cues.

√ Schedule pleasurable activities that engage all of your senses.

√ Explore new hobbies or interests that you are passionate about.

Extrovert

- What? You may be thinking, "How can this be a problem?" If you are a social butterfly, socializing typically involves food and sometimes alcohol. Alcohol has a tendency to lower your level of self-control when it comes to food choices, especially if you have been operating under restraint.

- Celebrating often involves pleasure-based eating or restaurant eating (large portions and lack of focus on fullness cues).

- Exposure to multiple food cues.

- You may allow stress to accumulate due to a busy social calendar, so less time is allotted for exercise or meal planning.

Strategies:

√ Have a plan: View your week ahead; balance nutrition and calories in the meals and on the days that you are at home and can be more in control of your choices.

√ "Mindful eating" and "eating with awareness": you can still try to do this when you are in a public setting.

√ Eat a small snack (protein and fiber combination) before you go out.

√ Socialize without the focus being on food.

√ Schedule time for stress management and self-care.

√ Exercising with a friend or going to a gym or fitness class will likely increase your motivation, as it can feel like social time.

Do You Practice "Restrained Eating"?

Most chronic dieters fit into this style of eating: chronically holding themselves back from eating how much/what they really want; and ignoring internal cues for hunger and relying on external rules for control. Staying in control of eating depends upon ability to remain calm and rational. Restrained eating puts you at risk for over-eating if you let your guard down or you become disinhibited (Herman and Polivy, 1975).

Options for dealing with this style of dieting/eating include:

1) Be aware of and plan for the most common disinhibitors:
   - Deprivation: keeping calories too low or not allowing favorite foods in moderation.
   - Fatigue and negative emotions.

- Alcohol.
- Breaking a "diet" rule: going over allotted calories or eating a forbidden food.
- Social situations: implies that it is not "business as usual," others are eating whatever they want, may feel left out, and multiple food cues are present.

Or,

2) Let go of this type of restrictive/all or none pattern and embrace balance: "Tier Approach," "planning and compensating," and Plan B.

Feeding Body • Mind • Soul • Spirit (Is there a void?)

The inner *glow* is about the other aspects of our lives and how fulfilled you are in those areas. Think of the *glow* that comes when you are walking in your truth, being authentic, and at peace with who you are. Think of the *glow* that comes after physical activity, when you have engaged your body in movement. Think of the *glow* of pregnancy or how you feel when you are gazing at your beloved child. Reflect back on the *glow* you have when you are falling in love, or feel deeply connected in a long-term relationship or friendship. Think of the *glow* you have when you truly love the work you do, whether it is a career, involvement in community or taking care of family. Think of the *glow* you feel when you have a spiritual experience or are surrounded by nature.

The *glow approach* goes beyond balancing calories; it's about balancing the type of food with which you nourish yourself and about creating balance in your whole life.

- **Nourishing Relationships**
- **Connecting to Community, Career and Spirituality**

Nourishing Relationships

Enjoying close interpersonal relationships is consistently related to happiness and life satisfaction. If you are not able to derive satisfaction and comfort through interactions with others, you may turn to food for solace. Food is a predictable, pleasurable, fulfilling experience.

When you are falling in love, your body produces a cocktail of feel good chemicals including oxytocin (bonding), dopamine, serotonin, norepinephrine, vasopressin, cortisol, and phenylethylamine.

Historically, women have been encouraged to seek their sense of self through relationships.

This isn't problematic if the relationship is healthy and reciprocal and/or she has other avenues of self-identity/self-worth to choose from. Problems may arise if she feels overly responsible for maintaining the relationship or is concerned about keeping harmony in the relationship at the expense of self. If there is a lack of intimacy or nurturance, food can fill that void.

Be honest with yourself about what your level of need is: do you want more or deeper connections with people? Do you have a relationship that allows you to feel safe enough to talk about real issues and be yourself?

_____

_____

_____

_____

_____

_____

_____

_____

Obsessing about food and weight can keep you from realistically assessing the relationship you are in:

- Does the relationship diminish your self-worth or does it build you up?

- Do you feel listened to, appreciated, validated, and loved?

- Do you have a voice, are your needs being met, and can you be authentic?

- Are you treated with respect or is there any type of abuse in the relationship?

- Does spouse/partner have any type of addictive disorder? Sometimes there is an unspoken quid pro quo, "I won't bug you about your problem and you won't bug me about mine...or, "If you are going to do that, then I am going to do this."

- Are you ambivalent about the relationship but don't know how to assert yourself or have the courage to leave?

- Do you think losing weight will give you the confidence to leave the relationship, yet you self-sabotage by gaining more weight?

If you are afraid of physical or emotional intimacy, you may protect yourself with weight, or isolate with food, or use weight as the excuse to isolate. A relationship with food may be a substitute for a relationship with people.

- Do you struggle with establishing relationships?
- Are you afraid that if other people really know you that they won't like you?
- Are you so fearful of being rejected that you do not let anyone get close to you?
- Are you masking feelings of isolation by filling the void with food?

_____

_____

_____

_____

_____

You may have learned unhealthy patterns of relating to others in your family-of-origin, although the family environment is not the only social setting where there may have been negative relational experiences. Your peer relationships and dating partners can also be formative templates and set the stage for re-enacting these patterns in present day relationships. We often are attracted to what is familiar, or to traits that are opposite of us to provide balance.

Exploring the purpose of food/weight in your relationship

If you are in a healthy relationship, food/weight may not be an issue. Subtle factors may include: enjoying going out to eat together or cooking/baking may be a part of your pleasurable experiences you enjoy together, or spouse may be a "food buddy" and engage in the eating behavior with you.

_____

_____

_____

What are the real issues that need to be addressed in the relationship and what is stopping

you from addressing them . . . fear, lack of skills? _____

_____

_____

_____

What feelings are you "stuffing" (passive or safe way of dealing with feelings) with food and why can't they be expressed directly? _____

_____

_____

Are you gaining weight to avoid intimacy?

- Trust issues in relationship
- Unresolved sexuality issues
- Unresolved sexual abuse issues
- Passive-aggressive attempt to punish spouse for affair, addiction, or being a workaholic?

_____

_____

_____

_____

Alternative Coping Strategies

√ Assess the quality of your relationships, especially if you feel lonely when you are around them.

√ You can't change other people; you can only change your response.

√ Nurturance may not come to you automatically. It is okay to admit that you need it and ask for it.

√ Learn to detach from others overreaction to you; don't personalize what isn't yours.

√ How can you assert/protect yourself without eating/using weight? You may benefit from Assertiveness training, including limit and boundary setting.

√ What you crave is deeper nourishment; get your nurturance from people, not food. When you learn to get your needs met through people, you won't have to fill that void with food.

√ It may be time to cultivate new or deeper relationships. True intimacy without wearing a mask is a relationship that allows you to be yourself and to feel safe enough to talk about real issues.

Connecting with Community, Career, and Spirituality

If you find yourself eating because you're bored, lonely, or trying to fill a void, it may be helpful to assess the other avenues of connecting with others and having purpose and meaning in your life.

> *"Too often we underestimate the power of a touch, a smile, a kind word, a listening ear, an honest compliment, or the smallest act of caring, all of which have the potential to turn a life around." – Leo Buscaglia*

Do you feel like you are part of a community?

- Neighborhood
- Work or school environment
- Church or other spiritual organization
- Team sport
- Leisure activity group

- Support group
- City and/or state organizations
- Political organizations
- Volunteering
- Other

Are there any changes that you need to make in this area of your life to feel fulfilled? ____

_____

_____

_____

_____

_____

Volunteering

It has been said that when one gives back, they end up benefiting as much as the person in need. Volunteering doesn't only facilitate social connection; it also improves self-esteem, lifts mood, and reduces stress.

Do you find meaning in the work that you do? (Career, occupation, education/school, primary caregiver/homemaker)_____

_____

_____

_____

_____

Do you feel like you need to make changes in this area?

_____

_____

_____

_____

_____

_____

A Word on Workaholism:

Workaholics tend to use work as the basis of their identity and self-esteem. It may be a way to avoid other issues. Workaholics may bury themselves in work in an attempt to suppress anxiety, anger, or depression, and may turn to easily accessible, quick-fix behaviors such as alcohol, drugs, or overeating. If the focus is on productivity then other activities such as exercise, relaxation, and even time with friends or family is not prioritized. The need for rest and recreation may also be minimized. Substances are easily accessible and don't require much time or effort. Eating may be seen as the only acceptable break. Individuals often eat while they work, thus contributing to mindless eating and food cue reinforcement *(see Modify Environment)*.

Spirituality

Your spirituality encompasses not only what gives your life meaning and purpose, but also your attitudes about life, oneself, and others. It includes the experience of being part of something larger than yourself.

If you feel empty and there is a void in your life, what you may crave is deeper nourishment. No addiction will ever fill the gaping hole that spiritual hunger creates; you need to nourish your soul.

Medical and psychological professionals are aware that religious and spiritual influences may often be beneficial in human health and healing. Larry Dossey, *Healing Words* and Herbert Benson *(1998)* report the benefits of prayer include:

- Stress reduction
- Alleviates anxiety and depression
- Lowers cholesterol
- Lowers blood pressure
- Fewer headaches

There is growing empirical evidence that spiritual approaches to treating clients are as effective, and sometimes more effective, than secular ones, particularly with religiously devout clients (Richards et al., 2006).

12-step programs rely on a higher power – someone or something greater than the self to conquer powerful addictions.

> *"God grant me the serenity to accept the things that I cannot change, courage to change the things that I can, and the wisdom to know the difference." – Reinhold Niebuhr*

Rick Warren D.MIN, Daniel Amen, MD, and Mark Hyman, MD, *The Daniel Plan*, utilize faith as an essential component of their weight-loss plan; instead of relying on your own willpower, God's power is the key to any transformational change in your life, including your health.

> *"Don't depend on your own power or strength, but on my Spirit" (Zechariah 4:6)*

What is God's intent for how we relate to food? Rachel Marie Stone, *Eat with Joy, Redeeming God's Gift of Food*, highlights stories from scripture: the "Garden of Eden," "the

Bread of life," "the manna story," "feeding 5,000," and "the Lord's Supper." Questions about dependence, independence, rebellion, trust, faith, and hope center around food. She references food as a living metaphor for God's sustaining love for his people. Scripture cautions us about gluttony, and also tells us to be generous and share our food with others who are less fortunate. "As Creator, God wants to provide for us, and He gave us our senses to enjoy the experience of eating. Therefore, it is more than okay to eat with the joy that comes from sincere gratitude, to the Creator who provides food for your nourishment." (Stone, 2013)

> *"So, whether you eat or drink or whatever you do, do it all for the glory of God"*
> *1 Corinthians 10:31*

Spirituality is a broad concept with room for many perspectives. In general, it includes a sense of connection to something higher than yourself, and it typically involves a search for meaning and purpose in life. As such, it is a universal human experience – something that touches all of us.

Those who speak of spirituality outside of religion often define themselves as spiritual but not religious. They generally believe in the existence of different "spiritual paths," emphasizing the importance of finding one's own individual path to spirituality.

Just as you have your own unique biopsychosocial history, you have your own spiritual beliefs as well. It may take the form of God, Christianity or any other religious practice, or a belief in a higher power, the universe, or nature.

What does your personal relationship with your higher power look like? _____

_____

_____

_____

_____

How would you like it to be? _____

_____

_____

_____

the *glow approach*

All major spiritual traditions include contemplative practices: meditation, scripture, or prayer.

> *"Be still, and know that I am God." Psalm 46:12*

As we look within ourselves and outward at our world we can be aware of the other ways He provides for our fulfillment:

- **Nature** and all the sights, sounds, and scents it bestows. The awe, relaxation, thrill, peace, and pleasure we can experience by being a part of it.

- **Our senses** can take in all that nature and man offers, from a beautiful sunset, to crashing ocean waves, to colorful butterflies, to aromatic flowers, to chirping birds, to walking on crunching autumn leaves, to the warm sun on our face.

- **Our Breath** as an opportunity to activate our PNS, our own "relaxation response" to deal with worldly stressors.

- **Whole food, herbs, and spices** with nutrients that can help or heal our bodies.

- **Our soul** as a conduit to connect our spirit with His Holy Spirit and have an opportunity to have a personal relationship with our Creator.

- **Joy** comes from the Spirit of God within you; happiness comes from the world. Happiness depends on circumstances; whereas joy transcends life circumstances.

Spirituality as a coping mechanism – transcending life circumstances with a spiritual perspective. I view it as the highest level of observing and making meaning out of the events in our lives. We can emotionally react to something, or we can utilize cognitive restructuring to respond rationally and factually. Sometimes, though, things do not make sense on an earthly level – loss, tragedies, natural disasters, trauma, etc. This is where spiritual perspective comes in. What does it mean spiritually? What is the lesson, the purpose, the "soul growth" or the dependence on, and faith and trust in our higher power all about?

> *"If you are in the world, you need to be in the Word."*

Spirituality is also a relationship with a higher being – God. Communicating with, feeling supported by, not feeling alone - those are characteristics of connecting with God. It is a feeling of inner peace, not having to deal with life on your own. If you let go of control, you can lift it all up to Him.

> *"Let Go and Let God."*

What is the connection between food and faith, food and spirituality, food and God?

- Is food filling a spiritual emptiness?
- Is food in some way being used to self-punish?
- Are you struggling with forgiveness – self or others?
- Is your self-esteem low?
- Where do you find your identity?
- Is your body-image negative?
- Are you lacking a support system?
- Are you lacking passion, purpose, and meaning in your life?

_____

_____

_____

_____

_____

_____

_____

Options for Expanding Your Spiritual Practice

√ Prayer

√ "Awe" experiences

√ Meditation

√ Spend time in nature

√ Gratitude journal

√ Forgiveness rituals

√ Random acts of kindness

√ Attend a religious/spiritual service

√ Read the Bible, a devotional, or other spiritual literature

Changing Your Relationship with Food

Have you begun to understand the role that food plays in your life? Gaining insight into your behavior will often make it less compulsive. Creating awareness is the first step of your transformational journey. You can't change what you don't know.

Your awareness record (AR) is a visual guide that helps identify your triggers to eat or overeat, minimize non-hunger related eating, and gain insight into your cravings. Self-monitoring is the gold standard for any successful, long-term weight-loss program. When you observe, record, and reflect, you gain the knowledge to help break old patterns.

When you have an urge to eat, your "bridge between mood and food" flow chart reminds you to stop, breathe, and reflect – What are you feeling? What do you actually need? It will guide you in differentiating between physical and psychological hunger (emotional eating, diet mentality, and environmental food cues). As you gain awareness of your triggers, you can begin to change how you respond. Your "recipe cards" will have a list of alternative behaviors for each of the "roles" emotional eating plays in your life.

Your awareness record will remind you to eat with body- awareness. What does your body actually need? When you associate what you eat with how it makes you feel physically and mentally, and how the food will nourish your body, it is easier to make healthier choices.

Your awareness record is a tool you will definitely want to use in the initial stage of this journey. Many individuals find it helpful to continue some aspect of it indefinitely (written food record, food- mood journal, or "mental" awareness and self-talk). Your AR is also a good tool to use to help get you back on track after a relapse.

Awareness Record *(See Appendix D)*

- The AR begins with a reminder of your goals and why you want to make specific lifestyle changes. When you are tempted by the instant gratification of a tempting food, you will be more likely to respond with goal-centered self-talk and alternative behavior if you remember your ultimate "why."
- Next, set a specific daily goal to challenge yourself with. For example, eat more vegetables – include two with lunch and dinner, or drink 8 glasses of water per day.
- When you are using the AR as a food record, keep track of your meals and snacks (any time you eat). There are columns for:
  - **Time** (to help discern how much time has passed since you last ate).

- **Nutrition** (portion size and nutrient content – Are you eating enough protein, healthy fat, and fiber to fill you up and keep you full? Are you avoiding sugar and refined carbohydrates to help keep blood sugar stable)?
- **Hunger/satiety** (begin to focus on internal cues for appetite and fullness – don't overeat).
- **Triggers or external cues**

    Physiology – tired, thirsty, pain, PMS, etc.

    Emotional eating – self-medicating, avoidance, filling a void, etc.

    Diet mentality (self-talk).

    Environmental food cues (sight, location, activity, etc.)

There is also a comment column to record additional information such as: how the food makes you feel physically or mentally, if you are noticing a pattern, or if it is an emotional eating episode and you are continuing your journaling in your food/mood journal.

- You can also track your water intake and schedule physical activity, relaxation, and other self-care.

- You are changing your focus on dieting to a focus on your health. The role of food is nutrition. Be aware of how food makes your body feel physically and mentally, and what your body needs to stay healthy.

- Your food/mood journal is a place where you can write in narrative style when you are having an urge to emotionally eat or after you have had an overeating episode.

Create a Bridge Between Food and Mood – Flowchart *(See Appendix E)*

This tool is designed to walk you through the steps of what to do when you have the urge to eat. It will help you to differentiate between physical and psychological hunger. These non-hunger cues can be managed by modifying your environment, challenging your self-talk or finding alternatives to emotional eating.

This flowchart is a reminder that you have a choice on which path you are going to take between mood and food, and that you are in control of your health destiny. You may begin to realize that you are lacking in certain areas (stress management or assertiveness skills), have a void (spiritual or relational), or are attempting to avoid any number of feelings. You may learn that your body needs more water, rest, activity, sensuality (a backrub, a warm bath), etc. You may decide that you need more hobbies or that you need to get more involved with family, friends, or community activities. You may begin to look for other ways to feel more fulfilled, experience pleasure, or pursue something you're passionate about.

"Recipe Cards" *(See Appendix F)*

As you become more aware of your emotional triggers and the role food plays to manage those feelings, you will be able to identify what you need to replace the emotional eating. You can create a "recipe card" that lists alternatives for your most common triggers. I will give you examples of some of the most common triggers, as well as options for alternatives.

Whenever we are emotionally overwhelmed, our brain tends to fall back into old behavior patterns. It is helpful to have list of alternatives written down and accessible, so when you have the urge to emotionally eat, your visual list ("recipe card") is readily available.

Food/Mood Journal

- What am I really feeling? What do I really need? You can use narrative style of journaling or the "column technique" to help you identify what you are feeling and thinking, and your plan of action.

- Example of "column technique" (especially helpful if you are overwhelmed with multiple emotions and multiple issues):

	Situation 1	Situation 2	Situation 3
Feeling:	• Sad	• Stressed	• Worried
Situation:	• Friend moved	• Work demands	• Finances
Plan:	• Journal	• Delegate	• Create a budget
	• Keep in contact with that friend	• Relaxation	• Talk with support person
	• Renew other friendships	• Self-care strategies	

You can obviously go into more detail. The "column technique" is meant to be a strategy that externalizes and organizes overwhelming thoughts, feelings, and issues. I call it being in a "tornado" state of mind, when you are experiencing multiple issues and multiple emotions. The feeling of being overwhelmed is generally a high-risk trigger for emotionally eating.

Steps to Managing Feelings:

1) Breathe

- Turn on your PNS (Parasympathetic Nervous System), by controlling your breath – slow, deep diaphragmatic breathing. *(See description later on in this chapter under the Relaxation Response section.)*

2) Identify feeling(s) and/or issue(s)

- Journal or column technique

3) How do I want to deal with this? (alternative coping strategy)

√ Emotional release (identify and externalize feelings)

- Emotional regulation strategies
- Journal or column technique
- Writing letters, poems, songs
- Social support
- Prayer
- Other

√ Physical release (decrease SNS "fight or flight", increase PNS "relaxations response")

- Relaxation strategies
- Exercise, physical activity
- Dance, art, music
- Other

√ Change perceptions (thought patterns)

- Cognitive restructuring
- Uncover core beliefs
- Monitor internal dialogue (self-talk)

√ Interpersonal skills

- Communicate feelings and needs
- Assertiveness and conflict resolution skills

√ Social support

√ Spirituality

√ Self-care

- Self-soothing strategies
- Positive affirmations
- Restorative practices

√ Other strategies or therapeutic techniques

- See stress management section
- CBT, DBT, MBSR, EFT, Acceptance and Commitment therapy, etc.

√ Healthy avoidance strategies

- Use when you are not ready to deal with the situation, but want an alternative to eating.

Stress Management Strategies

Coping skills can be divided into several different categories:

1) Problem-focused: managing the situation

2) Emotion-focused: managing the resulting emotion

3) Appraisal-focused: attempting to change one's outlook or perspective of the problem

The following list includes the most commonly used coping/stress management strategies:

- Identifying and externalizing feelings/journaling
- Emotion regulation skills
- Distress tolerance skills
- Cognitive restructuring
- Social support
- Assertiveness/conflict resolution skills
- Spirituality
- Physical activity/exercise
- Relaxation/mindfulness strategies
- Problem solving/prioritizing/decision making skills
- Affirmations
- Humor
- Nature

How can you use your strengths in new/different ways as a coping skill? _____

_____

_____

_____

_____

_____

Assertive Communication

When you can express your feelings and needs, set limits and boundaries, delegate responsibilities, and calmly resolve conflict, you free yourself from the distress that can result from suppressing your voice. Assertiveness is expressing your feelings/thoughts in a manner that respects yourself and the other person – speaking the truth with kindness.

Affirmations

The purpose of this strategy is to replace your negative self-talk with positive nurturing statements about yourself. Use positive, present tense wording. You may not believe those words at first; it takes time to integrate new perceptions into your self-concept.

What "old tapes" do you want to replace? How do you want to see yourself? How do loving, supportive people see you? Use the space provided here to get you started, but also write these statements on sticky notes and place them where you can see it, read it, and believe it – everyday.

√ _____

√ _____

√ _____

√ _____

√ _____

√ _____

√ _____

Humor

It has been said that "laughter is good medicine." Laughter lowers stress hormones and increases the release of endorphins (Benson, 1998). A person who laughs easily and "doesn't sweat the small stuff" has the capacity to handle the adversities in life. The act of smiling even lifts your mood. Try to include more opportunities for laughter in your life.

√ Rent a comedy

√ Watch funny pet videos

√ Hang out with children

√ Read a joke book

√ Listen to a comedian

√ Reminisce about humorous memories

√ _____

Social Support

> *"Find Inspiring people – Inspiring people are vitamins for our spirits. They come is all kinds of disguises and descriptions. If you open your heart to being inspired, they will appear."* – Sark, *Inspirational Sandwich*

Social support can provide a sense of belonging, acceptance, and validation. Involvement with other people can decrease loneliness, provide love and intimacy, and give a sense of meaning and purpose in life.

If faced with a problem, a friend can help by providing an alternative frame of reference (cognitive restructuring), a soothing word, or just a listening ear. Being involved in a support group is one of the behaviors that is included in successful weight-loss maintenance.

It is important to take inventory of your available support system and if found lacking, begin to take steps to rebuild it. Social support can include:

- Significant other
- Family
- Relatives
- Close friends
- Friends
- Acquaintances
- Colleagues/co-workers
- Community organizations (church, volunteer, sports, recreation, hobbies, etc.)
- Support group
- Professional support (counselor, dietitian, health/life coach, clergy, chiropractor, physical therapist, physician, etc.)

√

List your support network:

_____

_____

_____

Physical Activity/Movement/Exercise

- If you are looking for a magic pill...here it is. The benefits of being physically active go far beyond directly assisting in weight loss and sustaining a healthy weight. Not only are there a multitude of physical health benefits but also psychological benefits as well.

Physical Benefits (Callahan, 2002; IIN, 2015; Sternberg, 2010)**:**

- Deters Heart Disease
  - Lowers blood pressure (regulates adrenalin release)
  - Decreases cholesterol and triglycerides
  - Decreases LDL
  - Increases HDL
- Enhances the functioning of the cardiovascular and cardio-respiratory systems
- Enhances immune system
- Improves sleep
- Improves energy
  - Enhances oxygen transport throughout the body.
  - Increases the production of norephinephrine and regulates adrenalin.
- Alleviates constipation
- Increases bone density
  - May reduce or reverse bone mineral loss
- Improves the strength of connective tissues
- Improves flexibility, balance, and posture
- Decreases risk of some types of cancers: colon and breast.
- Lowers the risk of diabetes
  - Uses up glucose stored in the muscle cells, decreasing resistance to insulin.

- Eases pain associated with back problems, fibromyalgia, and osteoarthritis.
  - Enhances neuro-muscular relaxation
  - Stimulates endorphin release
- Alleviates menstrual cramps
- Stimulates overall circulation and brings color – that glow! – to your cheeks.

Psychological benefits (Scully et al, 1998):

- Increases self-confidence
- Helps relieve depression and anxiety
  - Increases levels of norepinephrine, dopamine, serotonin, and endorphins (all mood enhancers).
  - Enhances neuromuscular relaxation
- Enhances cognitive functioning (Foley-Henry, 2014)
  - Increases levels of dopamine and blood flow to the brain
- Can change brain waves from beta to alpha (relaxation)
- Increased alertness and energy
- Assists with physiological emotional regulation
- It's a great overall stress reliever

The Impact of Exercise on Body-Image and Weight

Because of its role in energy balance, physical activity is a critical factor in determining whether a person can maintain a healthy body weight, lose excess body weight, or maintain successful weight loss. It is definitely an area that needs to be assessed when you are looking at what lifestyle changes need to be made for sustaining a healthy weight and finding alternatives to emotional eating. Added benefits include:

- Improves body-image
- Improves mind-body connection and body-awareness.
- Improves body composition by maintaining and building lean muscle mass, while metabolizing fatty tissue.
  - Tones and firms your shape
  - Lose inches so decrease in clothing size
  - Increase in overall basal metabolism

- Increase in metabolic rate while active and for hours afterwards.

- Increase in fat burning enzymes.

- Helps lower blood sugar and decreases need for insulin, so decreases insulin resistance which ultimately assists in weight management.

Before starting any new exercise program, discuss/meet with your health care provider. Once you have clearance, start slowly and listen to your body. You may want to start with a personal trainer.

Exercise is a form of physical activity that is planned, structured, repetitive, and performed with the goal of improving health or fitness. There are different types of physical activity: aerobic, muscle-strengthening, bone-strengthening, and balance and flexibility activities.

Aerobic or cardio activity causes a person's heart rate to beat faster than usual. Brisk walking, jogging, bicycling, swimming, and dancing are some examples. Aerobic activity has three components: intensity (how hard you exercise, which can be measured by monitoring your heart rate), frequency (how often), and duration (how long).

Cardiovascular exercise also helps lower the risk of diabetes by using up glucose stored in the muscle cells, decreasing resistance to insulin. If exercise is regular enough to use up some of the body's fat stores, the whole body becomes more sensitive to insulin, enabling the pancreas to produce less and use glucose for energy.

People differ in how much physical activity they need to achieve and maintain a healthy weight; estimates are between 150-300 minutes a week of moderate- intensity activity (walking at a 4-mph pace).

High Intensity Interval Training (HIIT) is cited as one of the best exercise methods for fat burning. Alternate between a normal rate of speed for a small portion of time and then increase speed for half of that time. Another way to look at it is go at it hard for 30, 60, or 90 seconds, then decrease intensity twice as long. The total time of exercise is typically between 20-45 minutes, not more than 3 times per week. You can apply this to many different types of exercise (walk at normal pace for 2 minutes, then walk briskly for 60 seconds, or jog for 30 seconds, then walk for 60 seconds).

Muscle-Strengthening Activity

This kind of activity works on increasing muscle tissue. Resistance training, lifting weights, or using your body weight for resistance (pushups) are all examples. Around age 40, the average person loses about a half a pound of muscle mass each year, making this type of activity a must for rebuilding muscle tissue and increasing metabolic rate. Muscle-strengthening activities are recommended 2-3 times per week; make sure to allow 48 hours between work-outs to let the muscle tissue repair itself.

Bone-Strengthening Activity

This kind of activity (sometimes called weight-bearing activity) produces a force on the bones that promote bone growth and strength. Examples include brisk walking, jogging, jumping-jacks, and weight-lifting.

Stretching is a time you can focus on yourself and your body while you breathe and relax. Stretching not only reduces risk of injury but the improved range of motion will enhance your workouts. When you do weight bearing stretches you can help reduce the risk of osteoporosis.

Lifestyle Activities:

You can also become more physically active by increasing your lifestyle activities, aka movement. It can consist of taking the stairs, parking further away from your destination, or standing instead of sitting. It also includes hobbies, chores, and leisure activities: cleaning the house, mowing the yard, hiking, gardening, playing outside with your kids, tennis, golf... the list is endless. List your ideas for increasing movement in your life:

_____

_____

_____

_____

_____

_____

_____

_____

Increasing Exercise Motivation:

You know it is good for you, but if you are not already engaged in a consistent exercise routine then you may need a little help with your motivation. What are your barriers to being more physically active?

_____

_____

_____

What activities did you like to do when you were younger? Is there a version of it that interests you today?

_____

_____

_____

_____

_____

_____

Strategies for Increasing Motivation:

- Choose an activity you enjoy, the time of day that works best, alone or with a friend, indoor or outdoor, at a club or home, self-motivated or need coaching/instructor, etc.

_____

_____

_____

_____

_____

_____

- Use a day planner to schedule when you would be able to do the activity(s). If you are aiming for 3-5 times per week, then pencil in 5-7 different slots when you could be available for a backup plan.

Monday _____

Tuesday _____

Wednesday _____

Thursday _____

Friday _____

Saturday _____

Sunday _____

- Pair the exercise with something pleasant (walk outside and observe nature, watch TV or listen to book on tape while on treadmill/elliptical, do floor exercises while watching a movie)

_____

_____

_____

- Exercise with a friend _____

_____

_____

- Associate the purpose of physical activity with something other than dieting, so it becomes a lifestyle change (improved mood, more energy, better sleep, health benefits, etc.)

_____

_____

_____

_____

- Plan ahead: have outfit and shoes laid out for the morning or packed for after work; pack a banana or light snack if you exercise after work and are trying not to go home first.

_____

_____

_____

- If you're not in the mood for your full workout, give yourself permission to do a shortened version (if you planned on walking half an hour, tell yourself you can walk for 10 minutes. Once you get started you may feel like continuing for the original duration; even if you don't you will still get benefits: glucose metabolism, improved mood, increased energy).

- If you are aiming for half an hour per day of activity, and you don't have that amount of consecutive time, break it up into three 10-minute versions.

Restorative Practices

- Restore and Rebalance

Nurturing yourself (Self-care)

- Carve out some private time each day, even if it is only a few minutes. Designate a special spot with "your things" nearby (a favorite blanket, slippers, journal, magazine/ book/devotional, cup of tea, etc.) _____

_____

_____

_____

_____

- Do something relaxing (warm bath, yoga stretches, meditation).

- Connect with a friend.
- Connect with God.
- Spend time in nature.
- Take a 20-minute nap.
- Take a 10-minute walk.

- Give yourself a manicure or pedicure.
- Color in an adult (or child's) coloring book.
- Snuggle with your pet.
- Set boundaries, delegate, and say no if you feel like it.
- _____

Leisure

> *"Rest is not idleness, and to lie sometimes on the grass under trees on a summer day, listening to the murmur of the water, or watching the clouds float across the sky, is by no means a waste of time." – Sir John Lubbock*

Leisure differs from work, as it is a time when you are free from obligations, duties, and expectations. Nothing must be done or produced. This is when you get to just be: be yourself, express your interests, values, and personality. Leisure helps you to relax, unwind, restore, and rebalance. Do you need to find balance in this area? Need some ideas?

√ Arts and crafts	√ Computer activities	√ Individual sports
√ Adventure sports	√ Cultural arts	√ Music and singing
√ Building and repair	√ Community involvement	√ Shopping
√ Camping and outdoors	√ Dancing	√ Socializing
√ Cards and games	√ Entertaining and culinary arts	√ Team sports
√ Collecting	√ Gardening and nature	√ Travel

* _____

Nature

Being outdoors improves the body's sleep-wake-cycle signals. It also improves the secretion of melatonin, a hormone responsible for restful sleep.

Richard Taylor, University of Oregon was researching the fractal patterns of Jason Pollock's artwork and the mesmerizing effect it had on him and others. He realized that many of nature's objects are also fractal, featuring patterns that repeat at increasingly fine magnifications (a fern branch, clouds, trees, coastlines, mountains, seashells, a lightening strike). He surmised that this is one of the reasons why being in nature can be so soothing. His research found that the fractal structure of the eye matches the fractal image being viewed. After viewing a fractal image for one minute, his subject's brain wave patterns switched from beta to alpha (relaxed state).

√ Spend time in nature whenever you can.

√ Bring nature indoors with plants or flowers.

√ Incorporate time in nature with being active (walking, hiking, biking, water sports, etc.) and hobbies (gardening, golfing, skiing, etc.).

√ Look at pictures of nature containing fractal images.

√ Nature sounds can boost our levels of oxytocin which promotes relaxation and connection.

Water (sight, sounds, touch, and negative ions)

√ Take a walk or hang out by waterfalls, ocean, stream, or lake

√ Set the mood for a relaxing bath (dim lighting/candles, soft music, fragrant bath products - try lavender bath salts or vanilla sugar scrub).

√ Indoor fountain, backyard pond or stream

√ Sauna or a steamy shower

Aromatherapy

Our mind and body responds to the fragrance of an essential oil. That trigger sends messages to the part of the brain that controls emotions and mood. Closely linked with memory (both connect in the hippocampus) a certain smell or fragrance can transport us to a different time and place. Lavender has been used for anxiety and sleep. Lemon oil has been used to lift mood and peppermint to give a boost of energy. If you're considering aromatherapy, be aware of possible side effects and consult a doctor or trained aromatherapy practitioner before using.

Music

Either listening to or making your own music with your instrument of choice can stimulate alpha and theta brain waves and induce a state of relaxation, creativity, and insight (Colino, 2014). Music therapy has been used to reduce stress, distract from pain, and lower anxiety and depression. Art, dance, and other creative activities that are a channel for mindfulness can be used for stress reduction and mood enhancement as well.

Gratitude

Robert Emmons, PhD, a pioneer in gratitude research, suggests that practicing gratitude can lead to an increased sense of joy and satisfaction, lower stress levels, and greater resiliency. Expressing appreciation toward others triggers biological responses in the brain, including a rush of dopamine (feel-good chemical).

Keeping a gratitude journal:

• Practice looking for the positive.

- Choose a time of day to journal.

- Be specific, what made it special?

- Focus on people, not just things.

- Aim for 3-5 things that you appreciate/ are thankful for.

- "Count your blessings."

- "Pay it forward" as in "It is better (feels better) to give than receive." Gratitude – the experience when one unexpectedly benefits from another's altruistic act.

Have an "Awe" Experience

Awe:

- The feeling of being in the presence of something vast or beyond human scale, which transcends our current understanding of things (Keltner, 2013).

- An overwhelming feeling of reverence, admiration, or fear produced by that which is grand, sublime, or extremely powerful.

- It provokes a perceived vastness and a connection to something greater than us.

The benefits include:

- Increase in happiness or well-being

- Decrease in stress

- Increased creativity

- Expanded perception of time

- Increase in hope – Appreciate life

- Reduced levels of cytokines, a marker of inflammation that's linked to depression, along with other disorders (Stellar, 2015).

- In a nature-inspired awe – a calm and focused mind, a decrease in the stress response, an increase in Vitamin D, a connection to nature, and may sense the presence of a higher power.

- Transformative, life changing – especially with an intense religious or spiritual experience.

How to have an awe experience:

√ Experience grandeur in nature – the Grand Canyon, powerful waterfalls, a magnificent sunset, a majestic ocean or mountain scene, etc.

√ Watch and listen to a thunder/lightening storm

√ At night, look at the constellations against the black sky. In the evening, gaze at a spectacular sunset – a mix of clouds and vibrant colors. Wake up early to catch a glorious sunrise.

√ Connect with your Higher Power through prayer, praise and worship, or other.

√ Watch someone or something giving birth.

√ Scuba dive or snorkel (experience the underwater world).

√ View the world from a hot air balloon, airplane, or outer space.

Pet Therapy

Virtually any animal can provide "contact comfort," the calming effect of simple touch. Caring for, connecting with, petting, and even just watching animals (i.e., fish swimming in an aquarium) reduces cortisol level, lowers blood pressure, decreases anxiety, and increases levels of oxytocin (which promotes feeling of well-being, contentment, and relaxation), (Howard, 2014).

√ Spend time with your own pet.

√ Volunteer at a humane society; walk the dogs, pet the cats.

√ Go to a pet store and gaze at the fish in the aquariums.

The Relaxation Response (Parasympathetic Nervous System)

(Rest, Digest, Repair) aka Self-Healing

The autonomic nervous system is divided into the sympathetic nervous system (SNS) and the parasympathetic nervous system (PNS). Danger (stress) activates the SNS. When the danger is over, the PNS automatically kicks in. Because the breath is one of the only physiological functions that is both voluntary and involuntary, we can learn how to control the breathing process for the purpose of improving our overall health and well-being. By learning to use awareness and your mind you can begin to control your physiological reaction to stress.

Any restorative practice that includes diaphragmatic breathing will induce the relaxation response by activating the parasympathetic nervous system (PNS) via the vagus nerve that runs down both sides of the diaphragm. The relaxation response (RR) is a state of deep relaxation that decreases the physical and emotional response to stress by activating the

PNS: breath slows, heart rate and blood pressure decrease, muscles relax, and endorphins are released in the body (Benson, 1998).

If the RR is purposely sustained as breath is lengthened, then brain waves slow down to alpha waves, which create a calm, peaceful, reflective state of mind. Slower brain waves allow more time between thoughts, so you have more opportunity to choose which thoughts you respond to and what action to take (Kabot - Zinn; 1990, McBee, 2016). The benefits of being able to create a calm peacefulness through relaxation are considerable. When you have a daily relaxation practice, you will greatly reduce the effects of stress (via PNS activation) and indirectly support your weight loss efforts through the reduction of stress eating.

Numerous techniques elicit the relaxation response. They include:

- Diaphragmatic breathing
- Meditation (focusing on a word, phrase, or short prayer)
- Yoga, Tai Chi
- Progressive Muscle Relaxation
- Visual Imagery
- Mindfulness
- Autogenic training
- Self-hypnosis

All of these techniques share two basic components:

1) The focus of attention through watching your breath or repeating a word, prayer, phrase, or activity.

2) A passive attitude toward distracting thoughts and gently directing your mind back to your focal point.

> *"Then the Lord God formed the man out of the dust of the ground and blew into his nostrils the breath of life…" (Genesis 2:7a).*

> *Our breath is the bridge from our body to our mind. Breath is aligned to both body and mind, and it alone is the tool which can bring them both together, illuminating both and bringing both peace and calm.* – Thich Nhat Hanh, *The Miracle of Mindfulness*

Diaphragmatic Breathing

Stress triggers hyperventilation (quick, shallow breathing) which over time weakens breathing muscles (diaphragm.) Learning how to breathe correctly will not only decrease anxiety but if you relax, you may lose weight (decrease in cortisol).

√ Sit quietly in a comfortable position. Close your eyes. Relax your muscles. Breathe slowly and naturally.

1) Inhale slowly through your nose. Your stomach should expand, your chest should not. Breathe in slowly (4 seconds)

2) Exhale by pulling in stomach and let the air slowly, gently flow out through your nose (6 seconds).

3) Repeat the cycle.

   √ Note to self – if you are sucking in your stomach, you are not breathing . . . diaphragmatically, that is.

   √ Don't take in big, deep inhalations repeatedly as this will make you feel dizzy and may make you hyperventilate. Focus on exhaling for longer than you inhale.

   √ If focusing just on your breath is uncomfortable, pair the inhalation with thinking the word RELAX, and pair the exhalation with thinking the words LET GO. Relax . . . and let go.

Mindfulness: Paying attention to our lives, moment by moment, on purpose, in a certain way, and without judgment (Kabot-Zinn, 1990).

The philosophy of focusing on the present moment keeps the mind from ruminating about the past (regret, guilt) or worrying about the future (anticipatory anxiety). The directive is to intentionally use your senses to focus on a chosen experience, object, or activity while passively disregarding everything else; which means to just notice, be aware, without judgment. Accept that it (whatever it is) is there, but it doesn't need to influence you. Judgment can be useful at times, but we tend to overuse it. Acknowledge that you have a choice whether or not to let something influence you. It is learning to not get attached to the outcome.

Mechanisms of Mindfulness: attention regulation, body awareness, emotion regulation (reappraisal/non-judging awareness and exposure, extinction, and reconsolidation), sense of self, and compassion (Holzel et al. 2011). These benefits can directly and indirectly assist in managing food and weight issues.

How Mindfulness Helps:

• Changes neural pathways in the brain (neuro-plasticity): Mindfulness helps rewire unintegrated neural connections, to reintegrate different areas and functions of the brain which enhances the power of self-regulation (Siegel, MD. 2017).

- Changes (decreases) gray matter density in the amygdala (anxiety) and increases gray matter in the cingulated cortex (sustained attention) and the left hippocampus (memory and emotional regulation, thus, you learn to observe it and tolerate discomfort.

- Increases serotonin production (McBee, 2016).

- Formal practices
  √ Meditation
  √ Yoga/gentle stretching
  √ Walking meditation

- Informal practices
  √ Eat with awareness
  √ Pay attention to everyday activities (showering, washing dishes, etc.)
  √ Observe nature

- Mindfulness-Based Interventions
  - MBSR (Mindfulness Based Stress Reduction)
  - MBCT (Mindfulness Based Cognitive Therapy)
  - DBT (Dialectical Behavioral Therapy), Marsha Linehan
  - ACT (Acceptance and Commitment Therapy), Stephen Hays
  - Compassion/kindness/acceptance

- Radical Acceptance, Tara Brach

- Compassion practices, Kristen Neff

Meditation

Attention is turned inward; concentration is on a repetitive focus. Observe the arising and passing of thoughts, feelings, or sensations. Bring your mind back to the focus you have chosen. Develop an attitude of acceptance toward whatever happens in the process.

- Centering prayer

- Transcendental (TM)

- Mantra

- Yoga nidra

- Zen

- Mindfulness meditation

Any strategy that helps you to direct your attention inward will help you to increase your awareness of internal cues: hunger, satiety, and differentiating between physical and psychological hunger. As you slow your breath and your brain waves you will be able to think through your emotional eating urge and choose a more mindful response.

√ Stop . . . slow down . . . breath . . . be mindful . . . respond.

√ Metta Meditation:

May you be content – May you be well – May you be at peace –
May you be filled with compassion for self and others.

"I meditate on your Word day and night." Psalm 1:2

Yoga/Tai Chi

- Pranayama (control of the life force or breath)

Guided Imagery/Visualization

Imagery involves any internal experiences of mental images, memories, dreams, or fantasies. You can learn to direct imagery for positive results. The focus used in this method is the sensory experience. You can engage all of your senses to bring your attention inward, as if you were a part of the scene. For relaxation, choose a scene that is pleasant and peaceful.

√ Close your eyes and imagine each of the following. Which is more evocative?

- Sight: ocean, lake, mountain, garden, etc.
- Smell: fresh cut grass, roses or lilac, autumn leaves, etc.
- Sound: ocean waves, birds chirping, waterfall, raindrops, etc.
- Touch: warm sun on your skin, swimming on a hot day, etc.
- Taste: favorite dessert, tart lemon, coffee, etc.

√ Your Personal Visualization:

Sit quietly in a comfortable position. Close your eyes. Relax your muscles. Breathe slowly and naturally. Turn your focus inward. Bring to mind a scene where you would feel the most relaxed and at peace. Where are you? Who is there? What does it look like, sound like? Are there any aromas or scents? Do you feel any sensation, movement, or temperature on your skin? Passively disregard any intrusive thoughts, noise, or sensations; return your focus to your scene and relaxed breathing.

_____

_____

_____

_____

_____

_____

_____

_____

_____

_____

_____

_____

_____

_____

_____

_____

_____

Progressive Muscle Relaxation

By tensing large muscle groups, focusing on the sensation and then releasing the tension you will become aware of the ability to control muscle tension to relax your body. You typically will utilize all of the muscle groups, from head to toe (Jacobson, 1938). Breathing techniques and mindfulness techniques also can be incorporated. This is a great method of relaxation for individuals who have difficulty with sitting still and/or mental focus. This, along with yoga and tai chi, is considered an "active" relaxation technique.

Body Scan and Minis

It is helpful to set aside time each day (aim for 20 minutes) to practice a formal relaxation strategy. This allows you to reprogram/rebalance your nervous system. Many individual's pick late evening, prior to bedtime; as it can also help with insomnia.

Relaxation strategies can also be use in the moment, when you are feeling stressed or anxious. "Minis" use focused breathing (diaphragmatic) and can include short mantras ("Relax and let go") or brief versions of PMR or guided imagery. You can also incorporate aromatherapy (a few inhales from a vile of lavender scent).

You can also be preventative and use body scanning throughout the day to pinpoint if you are carrying any tension in your muscles or notice if your breathing is off. If needed, this can be a good time to utilize a "mini" and "reset" your nervous system.

Solitude

More than anything else, solitude is about achieving peace of mind, tranquility of spirit, and clarity of thought. Loneliness is when you are longing for something; solitude is about finding something.

> *"Solitude, quality solitude, is an assertion of self-worth, because only in the stillness can we hear the truth of our own unique voice."* – Pearl Cleage, *Deals with the Devil, and Other Reasons to Riot*

> *"One of the blessings of the old time Sabbath day was the calmness, restfulness, and holy peace that came from having a time of quiet solitude away from the world. There is a strength that is born in solitude."* – L.B. Cowman, *Streams in the Desert*

Solitude is your time to practice self-reflection. Be still; breathe. This can be part of your morning meditation or devotional time. Setting your intentions for the day: Who am I and who do I want to be; how do I want to live out my values, priorities, and goals? Be intentional about choices; not only with food, but also with your internal dialogue, your self-care, how you speak to and treat other people, and what gifts you want to leave to this world.

Chapter 2 Recap

√ Food Works! – No more guilt or shame!

√ Gain insight into how your past impacts your present behavior including food and weight issues. You can heal and change those re-enactments!

√ Listen to your "hunger," your inner voice.

√ Utilize Awareness Record – differentiate between physical and emotional hunger.

√ Understand the purpose of the disordered eating and the price you pay for those symptoms.

√ Create your bridge between mood and food; utilize "recipe cards" for alternative behaviors.

√ If food is filling a void, discover other ways to feed body, mind, soul, and spirit.

√ If eating is helping you to avoid something, utilize healthy avoidance strategies instead.

√ Build coping/stress management strategies.

√ Discover the role emotional eating serves to maintain your mask and shadow sides of your false self; rediscover your authentic self!

√ Utilize strategies that fit your personality style.

√ Engage in restorative practices: relaxation, meditation, etc.

√ Physical activity as a lifestyle.

√ Lifestyle changes – find your inner *glow*!

√ Change your relationship with food – transform your life!

Chapter 3 Summary

- Using Food to Self-Medicate
- Ruling out Mental-health (MH) conditions
- Strategies for Managing the MH symptoms that Interfere with Food and Weight Issues
- Understanding Food Addiction
- Appetite and Weight Regulation
  - The Role of Stress
  - The Role of Sleep
  - The Role of Ghrelin and Leptin
  - The Role of Estrogen
- Medical Conditions and Medications that May Impact Appetite and Weight Regulation
- Chronic Pain
- Healing Your Gut Microbiome

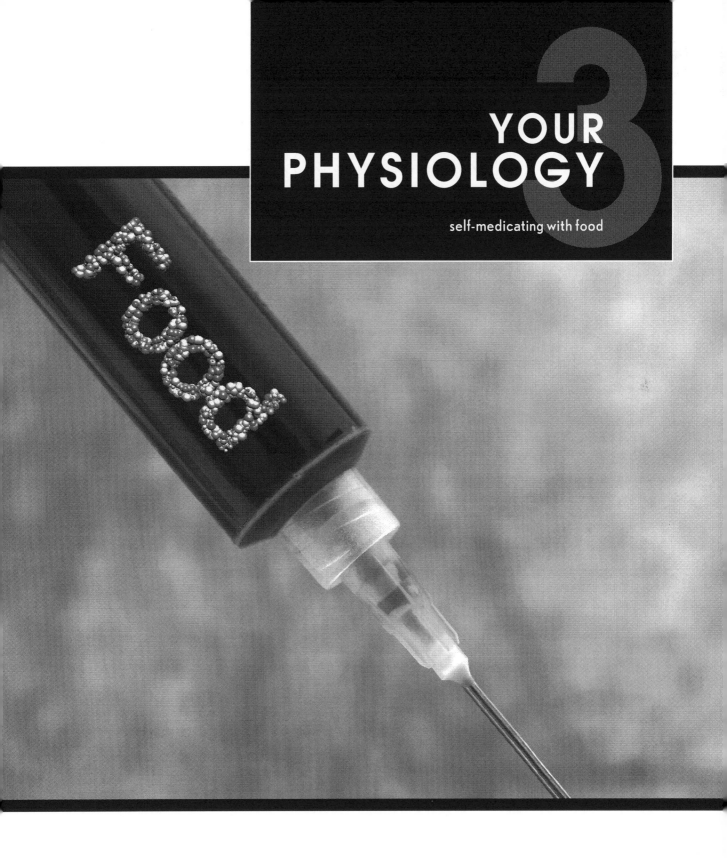

YOUR PHYSIOLOGY

3

self-medicating with food

*"The Lord your God, the Holy one of Israel,
has made you glorious."* — Isaiah 55:5b

It is important to be aware of your genetic make-up and to understand how it may play a role in your eating and weight loss difficulties. If you are unsure of why you are having difficulty losing weight or keeping it off, exploring your underlying physiology (mental and physical health) may yield some answers.

This chapter follows the Emotional Eating chapter because for some individuals, "emotional eating" is actually a symptom of an underlying condition or disorder. In essence, emotional eating is a conscious or subconscious attempt to "self-medicate" with food.

Food Works! Not only is the taste pleasurable and the act distracting, but food is mood-altering on a neurochemical level as well. Research shows that certain foods and lifestyle patterns affect powerful mood-modifying brain chemicals called neurotransmitters and hormones.

- Serotonin: Helps control appetite, satisfies cravings, and provides a feeling of well-being and inner calm. This neurotransmitter is released after eating carbohydrates. Foods containing tryptophan are precursors (building blocks) to serotonin.

- Dopamine and norepinephrine: Enhance mental concentration and alertness. These chemicals are released after eating protein (meat, poultry, dairy, legumes). These foods contain tyrosine, a precursor to these neurotransmitters. Dopamine is known to contribute to the pleasure-reward system that leads to addiction. Even the expectation of food (taste, smell, sight, thought) can increase dopamine. This sets into motion "drug" seeking behavior; for some people, the drug of choice is food.

- Endorphins: The body's natural opioid, which gives pain relief and pleasure when elevated. High fat food, sugar and refined carbohydrates increase endorphins, which work with dopamine to activate this reward system.

Emotional eaters often have underlying conditions that they unknowingly are attempting to "self-medicate" with food. It is important to rule out and treat this co-morbidity, as some of the symptoms of these conditions may interfere with losing weight and keeping it off. Depression, anxiety, bipolar disorders, obsessive compulsive disorder (OCD) , attention deficit disorder (ADD/ADHD) , post-traumatic stress disorder (PTSD), social anxiety, and borderline personality disorder (BPD) are among the diagnoses that are often seen in individuals who experience food and weight issues. *(See Appendix G.)*

In Amy Pershing's (2014) work with binge eating disorder, she identified the following statistics:

- Trauma/PTSD: 10x more common than in other eating disorders and 18x more common than in the general population. (This includes all types of abuse, attachment ruptures, and significant loss at an early age.)

- Depression: 15x more common than in the general population.
- Anxiety: 5x more common than in the general population.
- Bipolar: 5–7x more common than in the general population.
- High rates of ADD and autism.

Dr. Daniel Amen, *The Amen Solution – The Brain Healthy Way to Get Thinner, Smarter, and Happier*, through his work in the area of brain imaging, discovered five different brain patterns associated with being overweight: the compulsive overeater, the impulsive overeater (common in ADD), the impulsive-compulsive overeater, the sad or emotional overeater, and the anxious overeater. His treatment approach, including utilizing natural supplements, wholesome food, and healthy lifestyle, is individualized according to brain type.

Emotional eating is often a part of an actual eating disorder, such as anorexia, bulimia, orthorexia, or binge-eating disorder (BED). Compulsive eaters often identify themselves as "food addicts." It is not uncommon for there to be other addictive patterns co-occurring with compulsive/emotional eating, including but not limited to alcohol, drugs, or gambling.

The Connection Between Mental-Health Disorders and Difficulty Losing Weight or Keeping It Off:

Depression

This could include major depressive disorder, dysthymia (chronic low-grade depression), or seasonal affective disorder.

- Low energy and low motivation → decreased physical activity and lack of follow-through with food or exercise plans.

  √ Use a day planner to schedule exercise (having a written, visual plan helps increase motivation).

  √ Choose pleasurable activities that are not strenuous such as walking, yoga, and stretching.

  √ Enlist a friend to encourage you and exercise with you.

  √ Plan shorter time periods. (Once you start, you may feel like going longer).

- Decreased concentration and focus → difficulty with planning.

  √ This is a time when you may want to use Plan B food choices so you don't fall back in to old eating patterns *(see Sustainable Maintenance chapter)*.

  √ Make double recipes so you can freeze the extras to use on the days when you don't have the energy to plan or cook.

- Anhedonia (feel "flat" or absence of pleasure) → use food to experience pleasure.

  √ Have a "recipe card" with a list of a dozen pleasurable activities that you can do instead. (Have this already prepared since it will be difficult to be creative when you are feeling depressed. *Instructions for this can be found in the Emotional Eating chapter in the Awareness Record section.)*

  √ Have a soothing beverage picked out as an alternative.

- Poor sleep → disruption in circadian rhythm → disruption in metabolism and appetite hormones (leptin and ghrelin), and increased cortisol (increased appetite and belly fat).

  √ See section on sleep disturbance later in this chapter.

- Social isolation → increased exposure to food cues, decreased social support. Use food to "fill void."

  √ Reach out to trusted family or friends and let them know you need their help in staying connected.

  √ Utilize technology to stay connected if you don't feel like face to face contact or leaving your house.

  √ Join a support group or online support group.

  √ Spirituality *(see Emotional Eating chapter)*.

  √ *See Modify Environment chapter.*

- Increased appetite and weight gain (or decreased appetite and weight loss).

  √ *See Nutrition chapter* for healthful food choices.

- Carbohydrate and fat cravings, which stimulate the mood-elevating neurotransmitters serotonin and dopamine, and also endorphins.

  √ Use other methods to stimulate neurotransmitter and endorphin production including exercise, relaxation strategies, and others *(see Emotional Eating chapter under Restorative Practices)*.

  √ Discuss light therapy, supplements, and/or medication with health care provider.

Anxiety Disorders

- Worry thinking → defocus worry onto food/weight issues. Dieting is a socially acceptable and tangible replacement for other issues, so the problem/solution becomes, "I need to lose weight."

  √ Utilize cognitive restructuring to manage worry/real issues *(see Diet Mentality chapter)*.

  √ Utilize journaling or column technique to externalize worry thoughts and problem solve.

- Physical symptoms: agitation, restlessness, irritability, muscle tension (fight/flight response) → use food to calm (serotonin, endorphins).

  √ Physical activity/exercise to release tension and produce mood-enhancing neurotransmitters and hormones.

  √ Relaxation strategies to release serotonin and endorphins as well as promote more calming brain waves.

Social Anxiety Disorder

- If alone/lonely and bored → use food to comfort/nurture and fill the void.

  √ Cognitive restructuring is helpful to challenge some of the fears that are keeping you from engaging with others.

  √ Have a "recipe card" that lists ideas that you can do when you are bored and lonely.

Obsessive-Compulsive Personality Disorder or Traits

- Perfectionism → overly critical of self/body.

  √ Utilize cognitive restructuring *(see Diet Mentality chapter)*.

  √ Body-image work/healing *(see Body-Image chapter)*.

- Need for control → defocus on controlling food and weight.

  √ Gain insight into what other areas in your life that you do not feel in control of and what you need to do to change that.

  √ This characteristic may be governed by physiology, so addressing the underlying "OCD chemicals" may be needed.

  √ If you feel a need to count or keep track, begin to change the pattern from counting calories to focusing on the servings and types of food your body needs to be healthy.

- All/none thinking style → diet mentality: good/bad foods, on a diet/off diet, restrict/overeat.

√ *See Diet Mentality chapter.*

- Difficulty with decision making → difficulty knowing which is the "right" diet - may start and stop or switch around to different plans.

    √ The glow approach encourages you to design a plan that fits your biopsychosocial uniqueness.

- Rumination and need to act out behavior → thinking about food triggers an urge to eat that food.

    √ Use urge-surfing and mindfulness (see Food Addiction later in this chapter).

    √ Utilize Conditioned Eating strategies *(see Modify Environment chapter).*

    √ Utilize OCD strategies aimed at Exposure and Response Prevention.

ADD/ADHD

- Disorganized → Difficulty with keeping track of information related to food plan, shopping list, recipes. Difficulty looking ahead with planning meals, scheduling exercise and other self-care activities.

    √ Have one daily planner that you use to keep track of food plan, menu for the week, favorite recipes, shopping list, and scheduling exercise.

- Distracted → Difficulty staying on track with new food plan. Difficulty following complicated recipes that require too much time or focus.

    √ Have a written food plan; aim for a two week menu that you can rotate every other week.

    √ Choose simple recipes to use during week days.

    √ Use Plan B foods if feeling overwhelmed.

    √ Schedule physical activity/movement on a daily planner.

Eating is centering; overeating/ bingeing may stimulate dopamine, a neurotransmitter that helps with attention/focus.

    √ This usually happens in response to procrastination. Build skills that address procrastination and have a list of healthy avoidance options as an alternative to eating.

- Impulse control → Difficulty with delayed gratification and thinking about consequence of food choice versus immediate pleasure of food. Obese individuals have decreased metabolism in prefrontal regions that are involved in inhibitory control (Wang, et al. 2009).

    √ Make a list of your goals and what is motivating you to make changes in your eating habits.

√ Think about the negative consequence of eating that food: upset stomach, fatigue, rise in blood sugar, or negative health impact.

- Pleasure seeking → use food for gratification (dopamine, serotonin, and endorphin release). Food addiction and other addictions are common as a way to self-medicate by turning on reward pathways.

  √ Discover other alternatives that activate the other 4 senses and provide pleasure.

  √ Find healthy alternatives for the flavor/texture you are craving.

- Novelty seeking → easily bored, difficulty sticking to one diet plan, especially if it is restrictive and repetitive.

  √ Food plan: Change it up, make it interesting. After a specific amount of weight loss, take a break and focus on weight maintenance for a month (or even two weeks), then resume weight loss plan.

  √ Utilize the Tier Approach, as it allows variety in calorie/food options.

Bipolar Disorder Spectrum

- Impulse control → euphoria and racing thoughts, so not thinking through pros/cons of food choices.

  √ See ADHD

  √ Before going to a social situation involving food, visualize your plan of how you will handle food/alcohol choices.

- Pleasure seeking → over-indulging in food and/or alcohol to increase sense of celebration.

  √ See ADHD

  √ Focus on being mindful of the experience – without a substance.

- High energy/ irritability → use food to calm and center.

  √ Utilize physical activity and relaxation strategies.

Post-Traumatic Stress Disorder

- Trauma Response → heightened Sympathetic Nervous System, thus may use food to calm, self-sooth. At risk for other eating disorders, substance abuse, depression, and anxiety disorders.

  √ Use relaxation strategies.

  √ Mindfulness

  √ Yoga

√ EMDR (Eye Movement Desensitization and Reprocessing), Dr. Francine Shapiro

- Dissociation → use food to numb-out or center.

    √ Use Mindfulness strategies.

    √ Yoga

    √ Use "grounding" techniques.

- History of abuse → defocus onto body. May project self- hate onto body; control of food and body becomes symbolic way of gaining mastery/control. May use food to punish self (restrict/binge). May use body weight as protection.

    √ Resolve/heal underlying trauma *(see Emotional Eating chapter).*

    √ *See Body-Image Chapter.*

Borderline Personality Disorder

BPD is often a symptom of unresolved trauma – see PTSD. These individuals are at risk for other eating disorders, addictions, and mental health issues.

- Emotional dysregulation → use food to calm, dissociate, provide structure, release tension, feel pleasure, or to help with grounding or containment.

    √ Emotional regulation strategies/ DBT

    √ Physical activity/relaxation strategies/mindfulness

    √ Journaling and Cognitive restructuring

    √ Stress management techniques

- Poor self-identity → over-value body, so focus on dieting/scale to build self-esteem.

    √ Self-esteem building

    √ *See Emotional Eating chapter*

- Impulsive → lack of self-control in food choices or ending an eating episode.

    √ See ADHD

    √ Don't keep high-risk food in the house.

    √ Use Mindful eating strategies.

- Self-punishing → use overeating/bingeing as a means to inflict harm. (Emotional pain registers in the same area of the brain as physical pain.)

    √ Heal underlying issues

    √ Spirituality/forgiveness

- Rebellious → may see diet plan as something that you are being told to do, so may not follow it, as a symbolic way to be in control.

  √ Use Cognitive restructuring to help redo re-enactments from the past *(see Diet Mentality chapter)*.

  √ The *glow approach* is your plan that you design for you.

- Unstable relationships → Food is predictable; may use food for comfort and nurturance.

  √ Cultivate healthy relationships.

  √ Set and respect boundaries in relationships

  √ May need to build conflict resolution skills.

  √ *See Emotional Eating chapter.*

If you identify with any of the characteristics in these disorders, I encourage you to contact a professional to assist you in an accurate diagnosis. If these or other self-help strategies are not enough to manage your symptoms, please seek out additional support or referral from your health care provider; there are a variety of counseling strategies and/or medications that are available to treat each underlying condition. If you have been diagnosed with any of the following conditions, visit with your doctor or pharmacist regarding the medications you are taking and whether or not they have an impact on appetite or metabolism.

"Food" Addiction aka "Disordered Eating"

There are multiple points of view regarding "food addiction." Is it a true physiological addiction, an eating disorder, or just out of control cravings that are emotionally or physiologically triggered?

Most individuals who label themselves as such, typically describe multiple symptoms, including the loss of control over their ability to regulate consumption of food, preoccupation with when and what they will eat next, and having an expectation that the food will alter their mood.

There is no official definition or diagnosis for "food addiction." According to Mark Gold, Chief of Addiction Medicine, McKnight Brain Institute at University of Florida, food addiction is:

- Eating too much despite consequences, even dire consequences to health.
- Being preoccupied with food, food preparation, and meals.
- Trying and failing to cut back on food intake.
- Feeling guilty about eating and overeating.

These characteristics look like some of the criteria that are listed in the DSM-5 for binge eating disorder:

- Eating an amount of food that is larger than most people would eat and a sense of lack of control over eating.
- Eating large amounts of food when not physically hungry.
- Feeling disgusted with oneself, depressed, or very guilty afterward.

Most "food addicts" also identify with the behaviors listed under the DSM-5 criteria for substance dependence:

- Tolerance (a need for markedly increased amounts of the substance to achieve the desired effect).
- Withdrawal symptoms
- Uses more than intended.
- Tries to cut back.
- Spends much time seeking or consuming the substance or recovering from its effects.
- Use of the substance is interfering with important activities.
- Use of the substance continues despite known adverse consequences.

Research (INR, 2012) shows that people who are addicted to food tend to display many of the same characteristics of those who are addicted to drugs and alcohol:

- Use of behavior in times of stress.
- Common family history.
- Low self-esteem, depression, anxiety, and impulsivity.
- History of physical or sexual abuse.
- Obsessive preoccupations and compulsive behaviors.
- Experience mood altering effects from use of the substance.

Chronic consumption of highly palatable food can alter brain function in similar ways as the abuse of drugs. Research (Wang et al, 2009) shows that obese individuals and those who are addicted to alcohol or drugs show fewer dopamine receptors and or decreased production of dopamine. They may become more sensitive over time and need more of the substance that produces the dopamine (tolerance).

The foods that are most often included as having addictive qualities are high in sugar, fat, refined carbohydrates, salt, and caffeine. Some foods are intrinsically reinforcing because of their taste. Consumption of palatable foods induce the release of bliss chemicals (opioids and cannabinoids) that work in concert with dopamine to activate the brain's reward system, producing powerful reinforcement (Blass, 2008).

Cheese contains casein which triggers the release of casomorphins (feel good chemicals). William Davis, in his book, *Wheat Belly*, points to the gliadin, an opioid-like peptide (gluteomorphin) in gluten as being addictive.

Chocolate, without a doubt, is one of the most frequently named foods that people think of when they want a comfort food. Not only does chocolate have an appealing aroma and a seductive mouth feel, it contains anandamine (a cannabinoid-like fatty acid which triggers the dopamine reward system)), caffeine and theobromine (stimulants), tryptophan (a precursor to serotonin), and phenylethylamine (the same chemical produced when you fall in love), (INR, 1994). Chocolate also contains flavonoids (antioxidants) and a small amount of magnesium (calming).

Our expectation of food to give us a positive feeling or relieve a negative feeling will increase the craving for that food. Over time, neural pathways in our brain link the change in mood with the experience of eating that food (Volkow et al, 2008). Anything paired with that food can arouse anticipation of reward and stimulate dopamine release, thus increasing the craving *(see conditioned eating in Modify Your Environment chapter)*. Actions that lead to pleasure become imprinted in the brain and become habit.

In addition, alternating patterns of food restriction and bingeing contributes to reward dysfunction (change in neural circuiting) and an addictive pattern of eating (Cottone et al, 2008). This can happen with bulimia or restrained eating (ignoring internal cues for hunger and instead following self-imposed external rules) which can lead to overeating when the individual becomes disinhibited *(see Emotional Eating chapter)*.

What makes individuals prone to addictive behavior? Family history (genetics and role modeling) and an individual's own underlying physiology play a significant role in setting up a vulnerability. The individual may have a trait for high cortisol reactivity or variations in dopamine receptors (ADHD or depression) that make them more prone to addictive behaviors (INR, 2012). (Blum, 2000) described a syndrome called reward deficiency syndrome, which is characterized by abnormally low levels of dopamine D2 receptors, so individuals are more likely to seek out pleasure. Negative life experiences, including trauma and loss, also increase vulnerability *(see toxic stress in Emotional Eating chapter)*. Food and other addictive substances become a learned coping mechanism in response to stress.

"When we grow up experiencing the opposite of love – rejection, abuse –we become addicts in search of a feeling we have never experienced in a healthy way," says Bernie Siegel, author of *Peace, Love, and Healing*. Emotional pain registers in the anterior cingulated gyrus of the brain, the same area that registers physical pain. Just as opiates relieve physical pain, certain food can release endogenous opioids in the body and ease emotional distress.

Stress and Its Impact on Hunger and Weight Gain

Stress is defined as a state of mental or emotional strain or tension resulting from adverse or very demanding circumstances. Eustress is where stress enhances function, energizing or motivating you. Distress is where you feel overwhelmed and unable to cope with the situation.

Stress is accompanied by predictable biochemical, physiological, and behavioral changes. Stress may trigger emotional reactions such as anxiety, irritability, and depression. Physiological responses can include insomnia, high blood pressure, headaches, gastrointestinal distress, skin conditions, and impaired immune system. Chronic stress can contribute to auto-immune related illness, diabetes, heart disease, memory loss, thyroid/adrenal dysfunction, and some cancers (Kabot-Zinn, 2013; Weaver, 2015).

Behavioral responses can include low frustration tolerance and emotional reactivity/anger outbursts, poor impulse control, poor concentration due to distractibility, racing thoughts or rumination, negativity, decrease in sense of humor, and decrease in flexibility (either becoming more rigid in your position or becoming demanding or controlling of your environment or the people in it as a means to cope with threatened internal control).

The biochemical changes that occur in the body have come to be known as the "fight or flight response," or more aptly "fight, flight, or freeze." There are two pathways of this response: activation of the sympathetic nervous system and activation of the hypothalamic-pituitary-adrenal axis (HPA), (INR, 2012).

Sympathetic nervous system activation releases adrenalin which increases respirations, heart rate, blood-pressure, perspiration, and muscle tension. There is increased blood flow to the brain, heart, and working muscles. There is decreased blood flow to the intestines, an increase in frequency of brain waves, and changes in the endocrine, immunological, and autonomic nervous systems (Benson, 1998).

The HPA axis not only influences our response to stress, but also regulates digestion, immune function, mood and emotions, and energy storage and expenditure. The HPA axis is responsible for the releases of cortisol, which allows the release of glucose to be directed to the large muscles, heart, and brain.

Once the stress has ended, the body takes measures to regain balance by activating the parasympathetic nervous system — the "relaxation response," as coined by Dr. Herbert Benson (1998). Breathing slows down, heart rate and blood pressure decrease, and muscles relax. Hormones and neurotransmitters return to baseline. If the stress remains constant then these hormones will continue to be elevated and will have a negative effect on the immune system, food and weight regulation, and chronic disease risk.

Stress influences food intake indirectly via the biological changes that are activated by the stress response, as well as disinhibiting restraint with food choice and amount. Chronic stress elevates ghrelin (an appetite stimulating gut hormone), which appears to increase preference for high fat, high sugar foods.

Chronic activation of the HPA axis elicits the release of endogenous opioids, which stimulates cravings for high fat, high sugar foods. Fatty foods trigger the release of endorphins (endogenous opioids). If eating becomes a learned coping behavior to sustain opioid release, then consumption of highly palatable food becomes "addictive" (INR, 2012).

Chronic stress (chronic repetitive stress response) leads to high cortisol levels which increases appetite and carbohydrate (sugar) cravings. Cortisol is responsible for releasing glucose from cells into the blood stream, but since it isn't getting used to "fight or flight," blood sugar levels remain high.

Concurrently, cortisol inhibits insulin production in an attempt to prevent glucose from being stored. Insulin helps sugar get into the muscle cell versus being stored as fat. When cells are prevented from getting glucose they send out hunger signals. Cells become insulin resistant and the pancreas struggles to keep up with the demand for insulin. Blood sugar levels remain high so cells can't get rid of stored fat (Hyman, 2012; Ludwig, 2016).

High cortisol levels favor the increase in visceral (belly) fat, which produces inflammatory proteins called cytokines, which contribute to insulin resistance, diabetes, and heart disease, etc. Visceral fat increases the production of cortisol. High cortisol can impair memory, break down muscle tissue, and lead to chronic inflammation *(see Nutrition chapter)*.

Managing Stress

Stress needs to be viewed as a process that includes not only the stressor and our response, but mediators such as appraisal, sense of control, prior experiences, coping abilities, personality factors, social support, material resources, and other intervening variables. These variables account for the differences in reactions to stress. For example, a situation that feels challenging to one person may feel stressful to someone else.

Appraisal is the individual's perception or interpretation of the stressor and their options and resources for managing them. This is where cognitive restructuring would come in as an imperative coping skill for stress management. Self-efficacy is a characteristic that describes confidence in one's own coping abilities. If you don't feel like you have a repertoire of coping skills to select from, you will be more at risk to use food or other substances. How do you manage stress?

√ Stress management strategies

√ Time management strategies

√ Self-care strategies

√ See Emotional Eating chapter and sections on emotional regulation, stress management skills, physical activity, the relaxation response, restorative practices, coping skills, etc.

The Role of Sleep in Appetite and Weight Regulation

Most adults don't get the 7-9 hours of sleep their body needs to repair and restore. Research shows that if you are sleep deprived it can have a negative impact on your overall health.

Sleep deprivation also plays a role in obesity, insulin resistance, and diabetes (Naiman, 2015). Poor sleep (less than 7 hours/day):

• Interrupts your circadian rhythm, metabolism, and appetite regulation by increasing the production of ghrelin and cortisol and decreasing leptin production. Most individuals will notice the resulting increase in cravings the next day.

Sleeping less than 5 hours/day produces higher levels of endocannabinoid – a lipid that makes starchy and sweet foods more pleasurable to eat (INR, 2012).

Feeling tired is often a trigger for non-hunger eating. It may be that you think you're not ready to go to bed – go to bed! (Your body is telling you that you need rest).

If you have things to get done that can't wait until the next day, try walking up and down stairs for 5-10 minutes, or engage in another form of brisk activity to help increase your energy level. Green tea is less stimulating than coffee and also has a calming effect.

Sleep Hygiene Tips:

√ Resist eating too close to bedtime as the resulting increase in body temperature and metabolic rate will make it difficult to fall asleep.

√ Alcohol is both a stimulant and depressant; you may feel like it helps you to fall asleep but it usually causes middle of the night insomnia.

√ Caffeine typically takes 8 hours to leave your system. Even if you don't have any trouble falling asleep it may cause middle of the night insomnia.

√ Avoid eating sugar or refined carbohydrates before bedtime. It can cause a drop in blood glucose that can stimulate your body to wake up. Alcohol can do this as well.

√ Avoid foods with tyrosine (most protein) close to bedtime as it is a precursor to norepinephrine which increases energy.

√ Avoid screen time (computer, phone, e-book) in the evening as the blue light interferes with melatonin production.

√ Regular exercise enhances sleep; avoid exercising within two hours of going to bed.

√ Go to bed and get up at the same time each day.

√ Sleep in a cool, dark room.

√ Try foods high in tryptophan (bananas, milk) as it is a precursor to melatonin which is a natural sleep inducer.

√ Tart cherry juice is thought to stimulate melatonin. Pair with protein or high fiber to balance blood sugar.

√ Try sipping warm chamomile tea.

√ Use aromatherapy. Lavender is a relaxing scent.

√ Try a warm bath with lavender bath salts (contains magnesium, a muscle relaxant). The rise and then fall in body temperature simulates the body's natural response when falling asleep.

√ Set a relaxing, consistent bedtime routine.

√ Quiet your mind before bed: relaxation techniques, prayer, or light reading.

If you have difficulty falling asleep at night due to stress or anxiety, try writing down your worry thoughts and using cognitive restructuring to challenge them. If you are thinking of things you need to do the next day, write them out on a list. Once you clear your mind, it will be easier to focus on a relaxation strategy or write in your gratitude journal.

If sleep problems persist, you may benefit from cognitive behavioral therapy for insomnia (CBT-I). If your sleep is not restorative, you may need to be assessed for sleep apnea, restless leg syndrome, or other sleep disorders.

There are two problems that involve disordered eating primarily at night: nocturnal sleep-related eating disorder (NS-RED) and night eating syndrome (NES). NS-RED is characterized by sleepwalking and eating during non-REM sleep, while NES is defined as frequent and recurrent awakenings to eat and normal sleep onset following ingestion of desired food. Treatment options are available for both; a referral to a sleep disorder center is typically recommended for NS-RED, as it is also viewed a disturbance in sleep circadian rhythm.

Additional Information on Ghrelin and Leptin (Hunger and Satiety Hormones)

Leptin (the satiety hormone) is produced by fat cells.

√ Foods that help with leptin sensitivity: eggs and fish.

√ Foods that increase leptin are high in zinc (spinach, seafood, nuts, cocoa, beans, mushrooms, and pumpkin) and high in Omega -3's (walnuts, chia, flax, salmon, anchovies, sardines, kale, and summer squash).

√ Foods that increase leptin resistance include low nutrient, processed foods including soda, refined flour, and sugar, fructose, and MSG (so avoid or eat less of).

√ Fructose does not stimulate the production of leptin or insulin (so it doesn't help you feel full), and is not able to be used for energy. It is100 % metabolized in the liver and converted to triglycerides, promoting hyperlipidemia and insulin resistance.

√ Eating a very low-calorie diet decreases leptin.

Ghrelin (which signals hunger) is produced in our stomach and pancreas.

• Ghrelin levels are reduced for 3-4 hours after a meal, depending on the macronutrients that are ingested.

• How to decrease Ghrelin:

√ Get adequate sleep.

√ Decrease stress (cortisol level).

√ Heal your gut microbiome.

√ Protein deceases Ghrelin; be sure to have protein at breakfast, and at every meal.

√ Sugar does not decrease Ghrelin.

√ Increase omega – 3's.

√ Increase fiber and water at meal time to stretch the stomach walls.

Peptide YY (a protein that decreases appetite) is released by cells in the ileum in response to eating.

• To increase PYY:

√ Increase fiber.

√ Slow your rate of eating - wait 20 minutes before you have seconds to see if you are still hungry.

The Role of Estrogen in Food/Weight Issues

Perimenopause and Menopause

Perimenopausal changes are brought on by changing levels of ovarian hormones, such as estrogen. During this transition time to menopause, estrogen levels gradually decline, but they do so in an erratic fashion. Hot flashes, mood swings, and sleep disturbances are common and normal signs of perimenopause, which can last up to ten years.

Women between the ages of 35-55 have a 75% decrease in estrogen. As the ovaries decrease their production of estrogen, fat cells increase their role in estrogen production, thus your body protectively hangs on to these fat cells. As Debra Waterhouse, *Outsmarting the Midlife Fat Cell*, so aptly puts, "fat cells are looking out for our mental and physical well-being."

Estrogen is not just for fertility – it's also for your brain, heart, skin, bones and other organs – throughout your lifespan. Estrogen keeps arteries pliable, protecting against heart disease. Estrogen also helps maintain dopamine (focus, motivation, and pleasure) and serotonin, our mood stabilizing neurotransmitters.

Therefore, not only does estrogen play a direct role in weight-loss difficulties, it also impacts most mood related disorders via dopamine and serotonin levels. Thus, the urge to eat for "self-medicating" often increases.

Body shape typically changes with aging – from a "pear" (wide hips and thighs) to an "apple" (wide waist). Abdominal adipose tissue has more medical risks, including insulin resistance, which impedes weight loss.

From age 35 on, women lose ½ pound muscle per year and gain 1 ½ pound of fat, so will burn 40 calories less per day. Women lose 2x as much muscle mass as men. Metabolic rate is directly related to the amount of muscle mass we have. Therefore, unless you engage in activity to build muscle, your caloric needs to maintain your weight will decrease.

Thus, as we age, it physiologically becomes more challenging to lose weight – especially if you are a woman.

What Promotes Fat Storage (Lipogenic)

- Estrogen
- Dieting
- Skipping meals
- Sugar and refined carbohydrates
- Overeating
- Late night eating

What Promotes Fat Burning (Lipolytic)

- Following a low carbohydrate diet, minimizing sugar and refined carbohydrates
- Exercise, especially HIIT

Premenstrual Syndrome

Symptoms that involve food or weight:

- Sugar craving — (Luteal phase reduction in serotonin)
- Chocolate craving — (Luteal phase reduction in endorphins)
- Salt craving — (Estrogen mediated water retention)
- Increased body weight — (Water retention)

Medical Conditions that may Impact Appetite and Weight Regulation

Polycystic Ovarian Syndrome (PCOS)

PCOS is a reproductive-endocrine disorder that results in abnormal levels of certain hormones. In a polycystic ovary, there are many follicles, but they do not mature, and an egg is not released. Because the egg is not released, progesterone levels are too low, and androgen and estrogen are too high.

Many women with PCOS produce too much insulin, or the insulin they produce doesn't work as it should. Clinical indication may include obesity, insulin resistance, infertility, acne, and/or excess hair on the face and body. Sleep apnea and mood disorders may also be present.

Lifestyle changes:

√ Lowering insulin levels is vital to managing PCOS.

√ Daily exercise improves the body's use of insulin.

√ Decrease intake of foods high in sugar and refined carbohydrates.

Other Endocrine Disorders

If you have an unexplainable weight gain or increased appetite, there are other disorders that may include these symptoms as part of their presentation. A brief list of the most common disorders follows.

Thyroid Conditions:

- **Hashimotos** (an auto-immune disease, which causes inflammation of the thyroid gland): symptoms include fatigue, decreased metabolism, weight gain, and may increase appetite.

- **Non-Auto-immune Hypothyroid:** symptoms include decreased metabolism, weight gain, and may increase appetite.

- **Silent Thyroiditis** (can alternate between hypo- and hyper- thyroid symptoms): symptoms can include metabolic, weight, and appetite changes.

- **Hyperthyroid/Grave's Disease:** symptoms can include significant increase in appetite but no subsequent weight gain.

Lifestyle changes:

√ Increase exercise (may need 60 minutes most days of the week).

√ Decrease calories; choose whole foods that are nutrient rich and fill you up/keep you full *(see Nutrition chapter)*.

√ Decrease or avoid tobacco and alcohol (thyroid is sensitive to stimulants, thus increases symptoms).

√ Monitor caffeine and soy (may interfere with thyroid medication).

√ Discuss iodine amounts with your provider (your needs depend on whether or not your condition is auto-immune related).

√ You may need to avoid nonfermented soy (milk, tofu, soy burgers), as they are high in isoflavones, which are considered goitrogens (interfere with thyroid function – makes it difficult for the thyroid to absorb iodine). Fermented soy is okay (tempeh, soy sauce, tamari, and miso).

√ Raw cruciferous vegetables are also goitrogen, but cooking them helps.

√ Most specialists recommend a gluten- free diet, as the molecular structure of gluten is similar to thyroid tissue and your antibodies will go into the attack mode.

√ Avoid aspartame (may increase thyroid inflammation and antibodies).

√ Avoid sugar and refined carbohydrates, as they will add to your already decreased energy.

√ Add green tea (thermogenic food – increases metabolism).

√ Dr. David Brownstein, MD, *Natural Way to Health*, and Jill Grunweld, Holistic Health Coach, *Fire Your Thyroid* are excellent resources for which foods to include or avoid to help your thyroid or autoimmune disease. As always, consult your health care provider for your unique condition.

Diabetes and Insulin Resistance

√ See Nutrition chapter

Cushing's Disease (Hyperadrenocorticism)

• Weight gain (waist, between shoulders, face)

√ Exercise (avoid high-impact as bones are weak)

Other Medical Conditions

Hypoglycemia (low blood sugar)

• Increased appetite

√ Avoid sugar and refined carbohydrates.

√ Keep blood sugar steady with 3 meals and 3 snacks per day. Focus on complex carbohydrates that are high in fiber paired with lean protein and healthy fat.

Chronic Pain

Eating is a pleasurable distraction and a method of "self-medicating" with food. Fatty foods trigger the release of endogenous opiates (endorphins). Carbohydrates are a precursor (building block) to serotonin; sugar triggers a dopamine response (neurotransmitters that help lift mood).

√ Pain management programs

√ *Full Catastrophe Living*, by Jon Kabot Zinn, is an excellent workbook for chronic pain.

√ See Restorative Practices in the Emotional Eating chapter for ideas on natural alternatives to trigger endorphin release such as massage, acupuncture, relaxation strategies, etc.

√ Have a "recipe" card with a list of alternatives handy.

√ Utilize touch – hugs or massage (stimulates endorphin release and decreases cortisol).

√ Acupuncture also stimulates endorphins (our bodies' own opioids).

√ Use heat (warm bath, heating pad) or cold (ice packs), depending on type of pain.

Medications that Alter Metabolism or Increase Hunger

- Steroids (may increase appetite and cause water retention).

- Anti-depressants and anti-psychotics (may cause weight gain by increasing appetite and altering metabolism).

- Medications for the following conditions may cause weight gain by increasing appetite or metabolic changes: migraines, diabetes, seizure-disorders, auto-immune disorders, and mental health conditions.

- Contact your health care provider and/or pharmacist for further information regarding your health condition, the medications you are taking, and whether or not it/they play a role in appetite or weight.

Your Gut Microbiome

Your gut Microbiome is a mini-ecosystem that consists of all of the microorganisms, including good and bad bacteria, residing in your gastro-intestinal tract. We now know that gut health impacts not only our physical health but our mental health as well (Hyman, 2012; IIN, 2015; Liu, 2017; Park, 2014). The gut microbiome is also known as the "second brain" since 80% of the mood-regulator serotonin is produced there. It is also noteworthy that 70% of the body's immune system is located in the gut.

Maintaining gut health can protect against obesity, diabetes, depression, and gastro-intestinal disorders, as well as other diseases. There are many steps you can take to keep your gut healthy:

√ Probiotics (live bacteria that help establish good gut bacteria)
Found in
- Fermented foods such as yogurt, kimchi, kefir, sauerkraut, miso, pickled ginger, tempeh

- Probiotic supplements (Consult with your provider, as different individuals with different conditions require different strains.)

√ Increase fiber (feeds good gut bacteria)

√ Prebiotics (indigestible fiber that nourishes good gut bacteria)
   Found in
   - Onions, garlic, leeks, artichokes, bananas, honey, asparagus, chickpeas, red kidney beans, lentils, watermelon, grapefruit

There are also steps to take to avoid harming your gut microbiome:

√ Reduce stress

When you're stressed, your gut gets bathed in stress hormones, including cortisol, which decreases good bacteria and increases bad bacteria. (Bailey et al, 2001) found that early life stressors were also associated with changes in microbiome composition.

Cortisol has also been indicated in contributing to inflammation and "leaky gut" (increased intestinal permeability caused by damage to the mucosal barrier – the layer of cells lining the intestine). The barrier lets nutrients pass through to the blood but blocks larger particles and germs (which would create inflammation if able to pass through). These pro-inflammatory cytokines may be involved in the pathogenesis of certain autoimmune conditions and depression, and are basically indicated as the root of most chronic disease (Amen, 2011; Colbert, 2016; Hyman, 2012; Liu, 2017; Perimutter, 2015).

(Schmidt et al, 2015) found prebiotics to be helpful in decreasing waking cortisol levels, the probiotic lactobacteria spp normalized cortisol levels, and lactobacteria farcim decreased intestinal permeability.

√ Avoid processed foods. Not only does it cause inflammation, but bad bacteria feed off sugar.

√ Take antibiotics only when necessary (as indicated by your health provider), as they kill the good bacteria along with the bad bugs.
   - Talk to your provider about adding probiotic supplements if antibiotics are needed.
   - Milk, eggs, and meat have antibiotics in them unless the animals were raised antibiotic-free.

√ Alcohol kills good bacteria in the gut.

√ Coffee stimulates acid which causes inflammation

Chapter 3 Recap

√ Rule out and/or treat co-morbidity (underlying mental-health disorders).

√ You will have greater success with weight-loss and weight maintenance if the underlying mental health condition is stabilized.

√ Understand the physiology and psychology of "food" addiction.

√ Utilize stress-management strategies.

√ Get 7-9 hours of sleep.

√ Manage ghrelin and leptin levels.

√ Low estrogen levels make losing weight more of a challenge – increase HIIT exercise and decrease sugar/refined carbohydrate intake to compensate.

√ Be aware of medical conditions and medication that impact appetite and weight regulation; utilize strategies to compensate.

√ Manage chronic pain.

√ Heal your gut microbiome.

Chapter 4 Summary

- Cognitive Restructuring – Changing the Way you Think
- Common "Diet Mentality" Distortions
- The Tier Approach
- Planning and Compensating
- Understanding the Number on the Scale

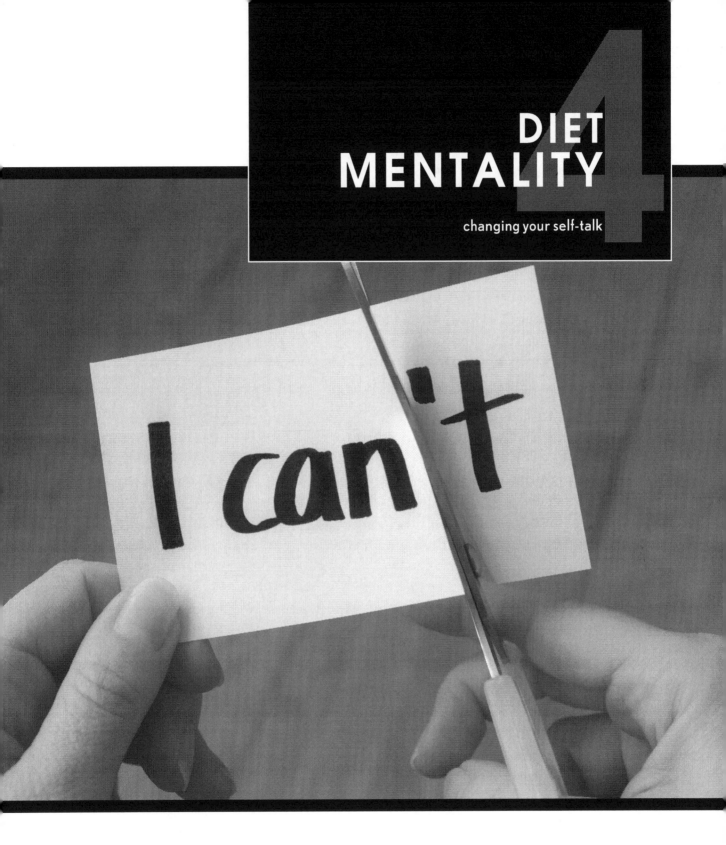

DIET
MENTALITY
4
changing your self-talk

"How wonderful to be wise, to analyze and interpret things. Wisdom lights up a person's face!" –Ecclesiastes 8:1

Does your internal dialogue promote and protect your health? Your self-talk can make a difference between self-sabotage and weight-loss success. You can take control of your inner voice. The first step to changing your negative voice is to be aware of your automatic thoughts: how you view your food choices, weight and body image, and other related issues.

There are common themes with the cognitive distortions (irrational thinking) that are present with "Diet Mentality." Change occurs when you begin to identify the distortions in thinking and replace them with rational, factual, and healing truths.

Evelyn Tribole, MS, RD and Elyse Resch, MS, RD, in their groundbreaking book, *Intuitive Eating*, were instrumental in bringing attention to the idea that there were other triggers such as "diet mentality", independent of emotional eating, that interfere with an individual's ability to stop eating even when full. The voices that they identify include the food police, the diet rebel, and the nutrition informant. They also put a label on the overeating that occurs before embarking on a traditional diet, "the last supper syndrome," which I include in my list of themes.

Dr. Phil McGraw's *The Ultimate Weight Solution* (2003), an excellent comprehensive review of the obesity literature presented in Dr. Phil style, also highlights the importance of awareness of our thought patterns. This includes the idea of self-responsibility under the construct of locus of control. Internal locus of control means you take ownership for the outcome of your life, are accountable for the decisions you make, and are in control of your destiny. You also have within you or access to resources to help you take charge of your life. External locus of control means that you feel that circumstances outside of your control guide your destiny and that you feel powerless to change things. This usually comes from experiencing "learned helplessness" in childhood, where there were truly no choices or options.

You **can** challenge and change your thinking patterns and the underlying core beliefs that influence them. Learn to eat without guilt or shame; it is not a moral issue. You deserve to eat and nourish your body with nutrition.

The *glow approach* helps you identify what negative thinking patterns need to be challenged, including all-or-none thinking, the critic, the ghost, "I deserve it", "It's not business as usual", the camel, waste or waist, and the last supper.

The Strategy:

Cognitive Restructuring: Changing the way you think (Beck, 1976)

Our emotional response to a situation stems mainly from how we perceive or interpret that situation, not from the situation itself. Cognitive restructuring is a tool to help you monitor your internal dialogue (self-talk), identify distortions in thinking, and replace the automatic negative thought with truth, facts, a neutral response, or a healthy compassionate voice. You can take this tool even deeper by adding the practice of mindfulness, which focuses on noticing the thought or situation without judgment.

Cognitive restructuring can be used to challenge any aspect of your belief system: your attributes about food, weight, and body-image; assumptions about self-worth/identity; values related to performance and expectations; and attitudes and beliefs received from your family, culture, or others. This coping strategy can help raise your self-esteem, motivate assertiveness, manage anxiety/depression/anger, redefine and heal past issues, and extinguish "diet mentality."

If you have a strong emotional reaction to an event, use the emotion as a signal to assess your thought process. See whether or not you are viewing the situation accurately. What are the facts that support the automatic response compared to the facts that support the alternative response? Most distortions in thinking fall into one of the following categories:

All or None Thinking: You see things in black or white categories. If your performance falls short of perfect, you see yourself as a total failure.

Overgeneralization: You see a single negative event as a never-ending pattern of defeat.

Mental Filter: You pick out a single negative detail and dwell on it exclusively, so your vision of all reality becomes blurred.

Disqualifying the Positive: You reject positive experiences by insisting that they don't count for some reason, typically because it isn't consistent with your core beliefs.

Jumping to Conclusions: You make a negative interpretation, focusing on aspects that support your core beliefs, even though there are no definite facts that support your conclusion.

Catastrophizing or Minimizing: You exaggerate the importance of things in a negative direction (worry thinking), or you shrink the importance of something (like your own desirable qualities).

Emotional Reasoning: You assume that your negative emotions reflect the way things really are. "I feel it, therefore it must be true." It may just be an underlying chemical imbalance (PMS, depression, anxiety, etc.), or you are looking at the present through past-colored glasses (re-enactment).

Should Statements: You try to motivate self and/or others with absolutes. The emotional response is guilt, low self-worth, or frustration. Expectations for self or others may be unrealistically high.

Labeling and Mislabeling: Instead of describing the error or behavior, you attach a negative label to yourself or another person. Mislabeling involves describing the event with emotionally loaded language (the intensity/volume of the reaction doesn't match the crime).

Personalization: You see yourself as the cause of some negative external event, which, in fact, you were not primarily responsible for.

Projection: You believe someone is thinking something about you, but you are actually thinking it about yourself. You may also have difficulty owning something about yourself, so you are seeing it in another person.

> *"The real voyage of discovery consists not in seeking new landscapes, but in having new eyes."* – Marcel Proust

Cognitive Restructuring Guide

It may be helpful to get your thoughts out of your head and onto paper. This coping strategy not only provides an emotional release, but it also helps you be more objective as you analyze the situation.

1) Describe the situation or event that is upsetting you. _____

_____

_____

2) What are you feeling? _____

_____

3) What is your automatic thought about the situation? _____

_____

4) What are the facts to support your interpretation? _____

_____

5) What is an alternative way of perceiving the situation? _____

_____

6) What are the facts to support this alternative view? _____

_____

7) How are you feeling now? _____

_____

If you are still stuck in a "What if" mode:

8) What is the worst thing that could happen if your original automatic thought were

true? _____

_____

9) How would you handle it? And then what? (Focus on the plan, not the worry

thinking.) _____

_____

Your thoughts and feelings about a situation often lead to a behavioral response. Thus, Cognitive Restructuring is a helpful tool in challenging the "diet mentality" that often triggers overeating.

Common Distortions with "Diet Mentality" that Trigger Non-Hunger Eating or Overeating:

All or None Thinking

This is one of the most common diet mentality traps. It is an extreme or perfectionist type of thinking. If your performance falls short of perfect, then you have failed; i.e., either on or off diet, good or bad food, restrict or overeat, etc. If you don't live up to your restrictive diet rules, then you go back to your old habits. This type of thinking makes you feel hopeless, and leads you to believe that there are only two options: perfection or failure. Extreme diet plans often set you up for this type of thinking if there is no option for flexibility built in.

Examples: You tell yourself you can't eat any sugar, and a colleague brings brownies to work. You eat one and your automatic thought is, "I blew it, I might as well have 3 more;" or later, "I have already blown it for today, it doesn't matter what I eat the rest of the day."

Two of the best strategies to respond to this type of thinking utilize the Tier Approach and Planning and Compensating.

- **The Tier Approach**

    This strategy is easily explained using calories, but you can also substitute exchanges, points, or food groups.

    Example: If your calorie limit for weight-loss is 1500/day, instead of fixating on that one number and being fearful of going over, use tiers with calorie ranges to allow for flexibility, not only during the weight-loss stage but also during maintenance.

    Example:

1st Tier	1400-1600	Weight- loss
2nd Tier	1600-1800	Slow weight- loss
3rd Tier	1800-2000	Maintenance

    (Calorie range for different tiers depends on gender, height, weight, and activity level.)

    - **Planning and Compensating**
      These strategies help you to balance your calories and nutrition within a meal, a day, or a week. It allows you to stay within your goals, but also have the flexibility to eat something that is higher in calories or less nutritious than you originally planned for.

    - **Planning**

      This strategy is proactive – looking ahead and assessing that a meal, treat, party, holiday, or vacation may not have the food/calories/nutrition that is on your weight-loss/health plan. You basically "bank" calories earlier in the day or week so that you have leftover calories to use later. This doesn't mean starving or restricting. Typically, if you choose lean protein, non-starchy vegetables, and some healthy fat, you will not only be balancing calories but also nutrition as well.

Example: If you are invited to dinner at a pizza restaurant, instead of restricting all day, over-eating the pizza, or not going at all, you can plan for it by balancing your nutrition and/or calories earlier in the day. So, depending on your biopsychosocial uniqueness, breakfast might include a 2-egg and vegetable omelet (200 calories); lunch may include an Oriental chicken salad, made with spinach, red pepper, peapods, cashews, mandarin orange slices, and raspberry-olive oil vinaigrette (400 calories). If you are aiming for 1500 calories, then 2 pieces of thin crust pizza and a side salad would get you there. If it is supreme thick crust, and you want 2 pieces, you may end up with 1700 calories. However, if you are also using the Tier Approach, then you are still within the (slow) weight-loss range – 2nd Tier.

- **Compensating**

  This strategy is used when you have eaten a food or meal that, during your former "diet mentality" days, you may have responded with "all or none" thoughts or behaviors. Instead of thinking that you have blown it and responding by restricting or overeating, you can compensate later in the day or the next by choosing lower calorie nutrient -dense foods.

  Example: You start your day with Greek yogurt with walnuts, chia seeds, and blueberries (300 calories). Your co-worker invites you to lunch and you end up eating a cheese burger and fries (1000 calories). Instead of thinking that you have blown it and respond by making poor choices the rest of the day, you can compensate by what you choose to eat for dinner. You may decide on grilled chicken breast or salmon with a double serving of steamed/roasted/ or stir fried vegetables (200 calories), so then you are still at 1500 calories. Or maybe you have already made lasagna, so you have a small serving and add a large side salad full of raw vegetables (600 calories), now you are at 1900 calories, which is the 3rd Tier, maintenance. You are still in control; and having the flexibility of a maintenance day or two can actually help you stay on your weight loss plan long-term.

Planning and compensating is a great way to balance calories and nutrition. Along with using the Tier Approach, your food plan can be modified to allow you to continue with your weight-loss goals, as well as participate in life!

The Critic

This style of thinking is triggered when you are disappointed in a choice you have made, but instead of labeling your behavior, you label yourself. This style is common in individuals who have low self-esteem or are perfectionists with unrealistic high expectations of themselves. This negative self-talk can range from being hard on yourself to extreme put-downs that could be labeled as self-abuse.

A new pattern is learning to eat without shame or guilt; it is not a moral issue. Remember, food works! It is not about willpower, it is about gaining awareness of what is triggering you to eat. Be patient with yourself; this is a journey of discovery and transformation.

> *Example: You eat a brownie, and your self-talk is, "I am such a pig. I am never going to be able to lose weight. I am such a loser." An alternative response would include a more compassionate voice that looks at your behavior but does not label yourself. Make an observation without judgment. Judging yourself harshly may trigger an emotional eating episode to numb-out how you are now feeling about yourself, instead of allowing you to examine the behavior and learn from it. "Slips" are an opportunity to gain greater awareness and they are a normal part of the journey. Thus, an alternative response could be, "I didn't plan to eat that cookie, but it's okay; I can compensate for it by balancing out my calories and nutrition later today." Or, if it was non-hunger eating, the response might be, "It's okay; what can I learn from this? This is an opportunity to explore what the trigger may have been, so I can make a plan for the next time." If you make a food choice that you regret making, use the experience as an opportunity to look at your behavior and what led up to the decision; change the old habit of putting a negative label on yourself.*

If this critical thinking style is a pattern for you, there may be some core beliefs that need to be explored and challenged. *(See Emotional Eating chapter.)*

The Ghost

I use this term to describe a voice from your past that you have internalized and let become your voice. It may even be messages from our culture, the media, or advertisements. The message is, "you can't have that... you don't need that...etc." When we are told we can't have or do something, we often respond by rebelling and doing it, even if it doesn't advance our greater good. We think we are taking control, but it is really pseudo-independence. An alternative response is to recognize the ghost for what it is – the past. Realize that it has no control over you now, unless you let it. You can respond with, "I can eat this if I want to. If I choose to eat this, I will eat it mindfully and not overeat. I am in charge of my food plan and I take responsibility for the outcome. If my urge to eat is not hunger related, I know I have a choice to explore what else is going on and choose other alternatives."

I Deserve It

This automatic thought often comes after a difficult day or maybe even after a celebration. It is using food as a reward.

Example: "I had a rough day on my job, I deserve this candy bar." You don't deserve to eat junk. You don't deserve diabetes. You do deserve rest, praise, a hug, or whatever else it is that you may need. "I deserve to eat this apple and be healthy," vs. "I can't have a candy bar."

It's Not Business as Usual

This type of eating occurs when it is not your normal day and/or it's difficult to plan or make what is on your food plan.

Examples of this are vacations, holidays, parties, or other times that are departures from your normal routine.

The automatic thoughts to this are often, "I can't stay on my plan, it is too hard to diet, etc." Granted, these are situations that make following a rigid, strict "diet" challenging; however, if you use the Tier Approach and Planning and Compensating, you can not only enjoy these occasions, but get through them and maintain your weight goals.

The Camel

This describes when you are eating a meal or snack and you are not sure when you will eat again, so you overeat to the point of being uncomfortably full. A healthy option would be to choose foods that have staying power and are slow to digest, like protein and healthy fat. Another option would be to pack a snack for later.

Another version of this is when the specific food is only available for a limited time, i.e., your aunt's famous lefse or a sister's rumcake. "I won't have this for awhile, so I am going to have more than one." One alternative is to have a piece in the moment and to eat it mindfully and ask for another piece to have later. Another option is to get the recipe so you can have it again, thus avoiding feeling deprived and overeating in the moment.

Waste or Waist

This describes situations when you feel like you must continue to eat the food, even when your internal cues are telling you that you are comfortably full because you don't want to be wasteful. This can happen while dining out at a restaurant or buffet or even at home.

> *Example: You are eating dinner and you are comfortably full but you still have some food left on your plate. It was already "leftovers," so you can't save it. Your automatic thought might go something like this, "I don't want to throw this out because that's wasting food." Using cognitive restructuring: "It's okay; my health is more important than a few dollars. Continuing this pattern will cost me more in health care costs, and I need to learn to eat intuitively." Or, "Would I rather waste this food or have this food on my waist?" You are not a garbage disposal.*

If you are at a restaurant, bring the excess food home. If it doesn't save well, then focus on the present moment – the dining experience. You also can share an entrée or order off of the appetizer menu.

The Last Supper

This type of thinking and behavior occurs before you start your "diet." You are thinking of all of your favorite foods that you are going to miss out on, so not only do you eat those foods, but you probably eat them in amounts greater than you normally would. The reality is that you are overdosing your body on unhealthy foods all at once. The calories you consume, if you add them up, may well be beyond the calories you are reducing in the first week of your "diet." This is another example of all or none behavior. You may want to look at a more moderate response. Example: if your plan is to reduce sugar, and you want ice cream before you start, your automatic thought may be, "I am going to get a large milk shake because I am not going to have this for a while." An alternative response could be having a small milkshake instead as it will be easier to compensate for.

What are some of your common automatic thoughts related to food/eating/weight?

Example:

Situation: *I have been working hard to lose weight all week and the number on the scale has not changed.*

Feeling: *I feel frustrated and hopeless.*

142

Automatic thought: *It doesn't matter what I do, I'm just going to go ahead and eat* _____.

How did this thought affect your behavior? *I had an overeating episode.*

What is an alternative thought, based on facts? *The scale is only one way to determine success. It is important to remember that the number on the scale not only reflects tissue weight, but also water weight, which is influenced by a number of factors including hormones, sodium, exercise, and even barometric pressure. Aside from the scale, I can look at changes in waist circumference, clothing size, body fat composition, and even more importantly – the lifestyle changes that I am making that will not only take the weight off but keep it off.*

(Hint – Our automatic thoughts are often emotionally charged short sentences that initially look convincing. But if we make our alternative thought into a full paragraph, adding calming, rational facts, we typically will change our mind and, ultimately, our behavior.)

Situation: _____

_____

Feeling: _____

_____

Automatic thought: _____

_____

How could/did this thought affect your eating behavior? _____

_____

What is an alternative thought, based on facts? _____

_____

How will this affect what you do next? _____

_____

Decoding the Scale

The scale…there are so many automatic negative thoughts associated with this apparatus. The Body-image chapter will address the pros and cons of utilizing the scale as a means to track your weight loss progress. For now we will address the common "diet mentality" reactions to an unexpected change or no change on the scale.

The scale is not only measuring your body weight (fluid, bone, tissue, organs, muscle, adipose tissue/fat, etc.) but it also is influenced by:

- The weight of the food and beverages you have consumed (so if you drink 16 oz of water, the scale will go up a pound – temporarily).

- The sodium content of your food (ham, soy sauce, processed food, etc. equals temporary water retention.)

- Alcohol consumption (dehydrates, so body holds on to fluid).

- The contents in your small and large intestines (until you have a bowel movement).

- Hormonal fluctuations (yep, that bloating is water retention – temporary).

- Strength training (temporary intramuscular water retention).

- Cardio exercise, humidity, sauna – anything that makes you sweat (temporary fluid loss).

- Glycogen (stored carbohydrates in the liver and muscle): This energy reserve can weigh close to a pound and it includes an additional 3-4 lb of water. You use up this glycogen store if you don't consume enough carbohydrates. When you resume carbohydrate consumption – you restore this fuel reserve along with the additional water. (That is why you see an initial drastic weight (water) loss on low carbohydrate diets and why the scale goes up so quickly if you go off the plan and eat a carbohydrate.)

The scale does not measure your health, wellness, or fitness. You may choose to use it as a guide, as long as you use it wisely, and not as the only means to measure your success. Move away from letting the scale define you or affect your mood for the day. Weight- loss progress can be measured by looking at measurements, especially waist circumference (which influences cardiovascular health), change in clothing size, and even by how you look and feel.

If you lost weight, what did you lose? Water weight will always come back – it is supposed to. We want to maintain our muscle mass; it is metabolically active (calorie burning) tissue. Exercise will help you lose fatty tissue and inches by expending calories and increasing lean muscle tissue. This change in body composition may not show up on the scale, but it will result in a smaller clothing size. The number on the scale may actually increase slightly (temporarily) as fat is lighter in weight but takes up more space, where as lean muscle weighs more but it is more compact and takes up less space.

If the scale is saying something other than what you think it should, then:

- Don't react
- Don't give up hope
- Don't allow it to affect your motivation or weight-loss efforts.

Instead:

- Do Cognitive Restructuring
- If the scale has gone up, and you haven't consumed an extra 3500 calories (per pound), then something else is going on.
- Review the list of factors affecting water-weight gain.
- Use other things to measure your progress for the week:
  √ Did you improve the quality of your food choices?
  √ Did you keep your portions in check?
  √ Did you eat, not overeat?
  √ Did you engage in adequate movement/physical activity?
  √ Are you making changes in your lifestyle:
    - Are you challenging your diet mentality?
    - Are you responding to environmental food cues?
    - Are you eating mindfully?
    - Are you choosing alternative coping skills instead of emotionally eating?

The scale is only a tool. If you choose to weigh yourself to help with self-monitoring, the following guidelines are advised:

- Do not weigh more than once a day.
- Weigh first thing in the morning, after you have used the bathroom, before you eat or drink anything, and preferably naked.
- Weigh once a week, typically at the end of the week, prior to the weekend, i.e., Friday morning.
- Interpret the scale cognitively, not emotionally. Do not let the number define your self-worth, your mood, or your activities for the day. You are more than just a number on the scale!

"And the Truth shall set you Free" – John 8:32, NIV

Chapter 4 Recap

√ What you choose to focus your mind on, is **how** you will begin to feel.

√ Be aware of your self-talk related to food, weight, and self-esteem

√ Use cognitive restructuring to challenge critical self-talk

√ "Diet mentality" is often a trigger to eat or over-eat a food that you haven't planned for.

- "All or none thinking" often precedes over-eating or bingeing.
- Use cognitive restructuring to challenge "diet mentality."

√ The Tier approach and "planning and compensating" are useful balance strategies, especially as a response to "all or none" thinking.

√ Never get on the scale without being prepared to use cognitive restructuring to challenge your negative interpretation of the number.

Chapter 5 Summary

- Master Your Food Cues
- Reducing Exposure to High-risk Foods
- Meal Planning
- Grocery Shopping Guide
- Tips for:
    - Food storage
    - Food Preparation
    - Serving
    - Eating style
    - Clean-up
- Spring Clean your Pantry and Refrigerator
- Bringing balance into your home environment

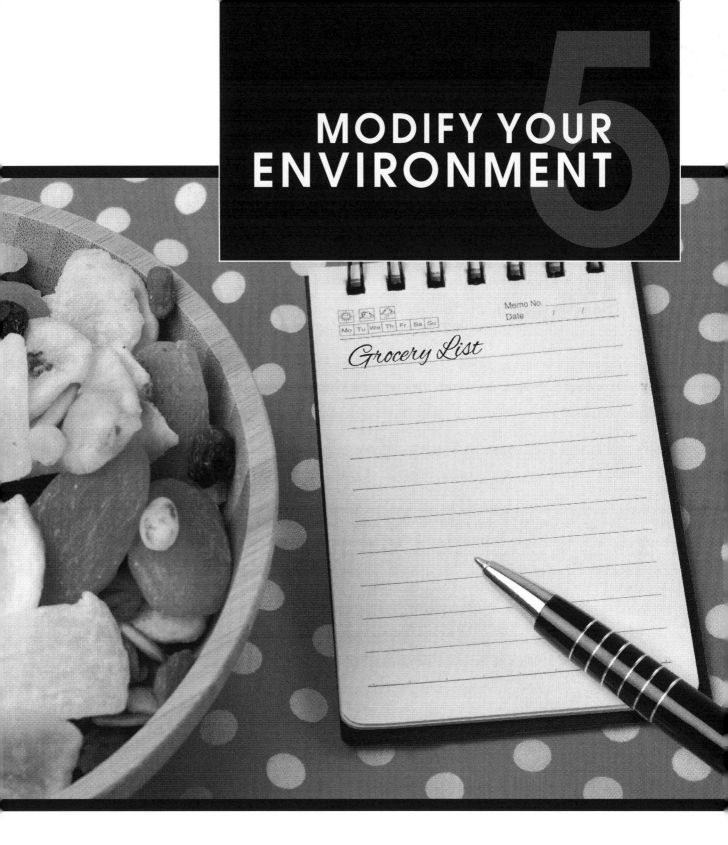

MODIFY YOUR ENVIRONMENT

5

Grocery List

"The only time to eat diet food is while you're waiting for the steak to cook." – Julia Child

It's not about willpower; it's about creating awareness of your environment and setting it up to be successful. The *glow approach* can help you arrange and manage your environment to support your goals.

Master Your Food Cues

Stimulus control involves learning what environmental cues trigger non-hunger eating, and then changing your response to that cue. Anything that you pair with eating becomes associated with food and can become a food cue.

- **Conditioned Eating:** Responding to food cues with eating
  Food cue → Urge to eat → Eat = Strengthens food cue.

- **Deconditioning:** Food cue → Urge to eat → Don't eat (substitute behavior) = Weakens food cue.

Common Food Cues: sight, smell, time, location, activity, people, thoughts, and feelings.

- Sight/Smell
  Visible and accessible food is often a cue for unplanned eating.

  √ Store food out of sight.

  √ Do not eat from the package (put food on a plate or napkin).

  √ Be aware of aroma coming from restaurants/theatre, driving
    past fast food joints, and going in to convenience stores.

  √ Avoid having high-risk food items in the house until you feel ready.

The aroma of food stimulates the olfactory nerve, which goes right to the hippocampus (memory center), which may increase the intensity of the craving.

- Time
  Be mindful of using internal cues for hunger versus the time on the clock (i.e., if you're used to having lunch at noon, but you just had brunch at 10:30, you won't be hungry by noon).

  √ Having set meal and snack times will help avoid "grazing" all afternoon or evening.

- Place
  If you eat in multiple areas of your home, those rooms become associated with eating and will trigger urges to eat.

  √ Limit eating to one room, sitting down, at a table.

- Activities
  (Watching TV/movies, reading, computer, studying, etc.)

If you eat and do any other activity at the same time, that activity becomes a food cue. Example: Do you have difficulty with grazing in the evening? Are you eating while you watch TV or read? If so, on a night when you are watching TV for several hours, you could be getting a continuous urge to eat because of the constant presence of the food cue, not to mention the food commercials.

√ Mindful eating: When you are engaged in another activity while you are eating, your attention is divided, so the awareness of what you are eating decreases. This means you may eat more to satisfy your "mouth hunger." This is not a time to multi-task. If you are going to eat, make that the event. Relaxing background music is okay, and it is even helpful at slowing your rate of eating.

- Thoughts/Images
  If you have a thought about food and respond by eating, you will begin to associate just thinking about food with needing to eat that food.

  √ Tip – use this as an opportunity to explore if there is an underlying trigger for the thought.

  √ Or try "riding the wave" – tell yourself that you can reassess the urge in 10 minutes. Meanwhile, get busy doing something else that is incompatible with eating. *(See "urge surfing" in Food Addiction section in Physiology chapter.)*

Thinking about food triggers hunger by stimulating the production of insulin, which decreases blood sugar; low blood sugar signals hunger. The expectation of food is enough to stimulate dopamine, the pleasure-seeking neurotransmitter. *(See Physiology chapter.)*

- Emotions
  If you frequently respond to an emotion (stress, boredom, etc.) with eating, then that emotion will become a food cue, and your automatic response will be to turn to food to cope with that feeling.

  √ Tip – Use your Awareness Record and journaling to create a bridge between food and mood. Discover alternative ways to manage those feelings.

How to Decondition:

- Thought Substitution

  √ Self-Talk: Tell yourself that if you resist the urge to eat (when you are not physically hungry), you will be helping to decondition yourself.

  √ Differentiate between physical and psychological hunger: What are you feeling? What do you expect the food to do for you?

- Urge Surfing *(see Sustainable Maintenance chapter).*

- Behavior Substitution
  √ Make a list of alternatives that fit the cue to replace the behavior of eating.
  √ Utilize "Recipe cards" *(See Appendix F.)*
- Avoid or eliminate the cue (i.e., pay for gas outside the convenience store).
- Sever the association of eating with the cue (i.e., don't eat while watching TV or reading).
- Change the circumstances surrounding the cue (i.e., plan to meet with friends in non-food settings).

Use your Awareness Record to help you identify what your food cues are, so you can begin to make lifestyle changes in those areas.

Reduce Exposure to High-Risk Foods

Plan a Menu for the Week

This will guide you in making a grocery list, which will decrease impulse buying at the store. As per Dr. Phil (2003), "You can't eat what you don't have in the house." (p.107)

Planning meals and snacks in advance will help avoid impulse eating. With your day planner, look ahead at the week's activities for you and/or members of your family. This way, you can plan accordingly, regarding who will be home and how much time you will have for meal preparation. Having a menu will also help decrease food waste, as you will be able to incorporate leftovers into a second meal or use produce in several different dishes.

Meal Planning Guidelines

1) Plan 3 meals and 1-3 snacks per day for 1 week.
2) Determine what your schedule is for the week. Use a day planner to help you visualize what nights you have activities; if you will have time to cook; or if you need to meal prep in advance, use leftovers, or plan a simple meal.
3) Your grocery list for the week is based on what staples you are low on and what ingredients/foods you need for your meals and snacks.
4) Planning ahead will help you have healthy choices available and decrease chances of picking up fast food. This includes planning your snacks in advance.
5) Simplify: If time is short during the week or you do not like to cook, then have 10 simple

recipes that you can alternate every other week. Choose ones with only a few ingredients and are quick to prepare. Utilize precut vegetables, prewashed and cut greens for salads, as well as canned and frozen vegetables/legumes/beans. Simple menus are often the easiest to maintain and incorporate into your lifestyle. *(See Appendix H.)*

6) Plan meals where you can incorporate part of the meal for leftovers for lunch and/or dinner, so you are only cooking once for two or three meals. You can also freeze for a later time. If you are buying an ingredient for a recipe but will not use all of it, think ahead to a recipe you can use it in. This way, it doesn't go to waste.

7) Most fruits and vegetables can be frozen if you aren't going to be able to eat them before they perish. You can use them later in smoothies, soups, and stews. Even cooked vegetables can be frozen to be used in this manner.

8) Utilize the weekend for experimenting with new recipes and enjoying meals that take longer to cook or prepare. This is also a good time to cook a meal or two with leftovers that can be eaten early in the week. This may also be a time when you prepare ingredients for weekday meals: cutting vegetables for a stir-fry, boiling eggs for snacks or egg salad, or making a homemade dressing or sauce.

Grocery Shopping

1) Always shop from a list to avoid impulse buying.

2 Your list should include staples that you are low on, food that is on your menu for the week, ingredients for specific recipes for the week, and Plan B food items. *(See Sustainable Maintenance chapter and Appendix H.)*

3) Shop after you have eaten, not when you are hungry. Chew a piece of gum.

4) Balance health and convenience: it's okay to use canned or frozen whole foods, look for pre-cut vegetables, bagged salads, etc.

5) Focus on buying foods that are located around the perimeter of the store. This is where you will find most of the fresh, minimally processed foods including produce, dairy, meat/fish, etc. When you are in the center aisles, search for minimally processed foods like nut butters; canned fish, beans, and vegetables; and frozen fruits and vegetables. Avoid impulse items at the end of aisles and at checkout.

6) Read food labels: Ingredient list is in order by weight. Avoid transfats and hydrogenated oils. Limit sugar and refined carbohydrates (look for 100% whole-grain). Be aware of saturated fats, sodium, nitrates, artificial ingredients, etc.

7) Buy whole, natural, unprocessed foods as often as possible. Buy seasonal (higher nutrients and less expensive) and local (know how it is farmed).

8) Know where your food comes from. Which foods are you going to buy that are organic, non-GMO, grass-fed/free-range/no hormones/antibiotics, through a Co-op or farmer's market, etc?

9) Don't buy high-risk foods until you are ready. Find healthy replacements that are similar in flavor, texture, and temperature. (See Appendix F.)

10) Avoid keeping unhealthy food in the house, as this will help decrease temptation. Keep a variety of healthy, yet desirable foods available.

Food Storage Tips

1) Store food out of sight; do not have food out on the counter or in bowls unless it is fruit.

2) Store problem foods in non-see-through containers in hard to reach places (in the back row of cupboard or behind healthy food in the refrigerator). Freeze treats for a later time.

3) You're more likely to eat the first thing you see, so keep cut up vegetables and other healthy snacks in plain view in the refrigerator.

Food Preparation Tips

1) On Sunday, look at what is in store for the week ahead. Pre-cook or chop ingredients, if it would simplify your work week.

2) Organize or prepare lunches the night before.

3) If this is a time when you graze, chew a piece of gum. If it is right before the meal, have some raw vegetable either plain or dipped in hummus or a yogurt dip.

4) Learn a variety of healthy cooking methods: steam, broil, poach, roast, grill, stir-fry, etc.

5) If you don't like a certain vegetable, try a different way of preparing it, such as roasting or grilling instead of boiled, from a can, or frozen.

Food Serving Tips

1) Avoid serving family-style (having food on the table); serve from the stove or counter.

2) Use a smaller plate or bowl. Visually, it will seem like you are eating more and will help you to be mindful of portion size.

3) Do not eat directly from the package, pan, etc. Put your food on a plate or napkin.

4) Sit down while you eat.

Eating Tips

Changing your eating style can help you eat less without feeling deprived.

1) Remember to always eat mindfully. Ask yourself, "Am I physically hungry? What does my body need, and how does this food make me feel?"

2) Start a meal when you are hungry (not ravenous); stop when you are satisfied (not overfull). It is okay not to finish all of the food on your plate if you are full; in fact, regularly doing so will help to decondition you to the sight of food being a food cue.

3) Eat at regular times. Do not skip meals.

4) Start your meal with a salad, raw vegetable, or a broth based soup. Drink 2 glasses of water with your meal.

5) Include foods in your meal that take time to chew, such as meat, vegetables, and salads. Try to chew slowly, putting your silverware down in between bites. It takes 20 minutes for your brain to get the message that you are full.

6) Include water dense and fiber rich foods to fill you up (vegetables, fruit, beans and legumes, oatmeal and other whole grains).

7) Include protein and healthy fats such as olive oil, avocados, and nuts to help keep you satiated (full) longer.

8) Leave the table and brush your teeth when you are finished eating; this will signal the end of the meal or snack.

Clean-Up Tips

1) Remove food from sight as soon as possible. Save it for leftovers, freeze it for a future meal, or throw it out – don't eat those last few spoonfuls. It is better to waste than have it on your waist!

2) Chew a piece of gum to refrain from picking at food.

"Spring Clean" Your Pantry and Refrigerator

If you are starting a new food plan/way of life, you can address this in a couple ways: 1) gradually by shaping – you select a series of short-term goals that get closer to the ultimate goal, which fosters success and increases motivation. 2) Start with a clean slate – out with the old and in with the new.

With shaping, you would focus on eating more of the healthy stuff and less of the unhealthy stuff. You might incorporate some of the food you already have into a meal with food you want to add to create a more balanced food plan. For example, if you have white rice in your pantry and you want to eventually switch to brown rice, then serve it with salmon and a vegetable stir-fry. If you want to start with a clean slate, it is time to spring clean your pantry and refrigerator. Donate or dispose of unhealthy food.

This is only a guide to get you started. This is where you get to decide what is on your food plan – what you want to eat more of/less of, what foods " work for you" for your health and weight goals, what your food preferences are, etc. You will want to modify according to your own unique needs, such as avoiding dairy, gluten-free, vegetarian, or soy-sensitive.

Pantry Staples

Steel-cut oats, brown and wild rice, kasha, quinoa, Ezekiel, sprouted, sourdough, or whole grain wheat bread

Dry or canned black beans, garbanzo beans, or other legumes

Canned green beans, beets, tomatoes, low sugar spaghetti sauce, and/or other vegetables or sauces

Canned or cupped fruit in water or natural juice, unsweetened applesauce, pumpkin puree

Canned or pouched tuna, salmon and/or other fish

Natural peanut butter and/or other nut butters

Nuts: walnuts, almonds, pecans, pistachios, and/or others.

Seeds: sunflower, pumpkin, sesame, chia, ground flax, and/or other

Extra virgin olive oil, walnut oil, sesame oil, unrefined extra virgin coconut oil; balsamic vinegar, apple cider vinegar, and/or other vinegars

Tamari, tahini, miso, wasabi paste, (you will store most of these in your refrigerator after opening)

Garlic and onion powder, pepper, sea salt, Stevia, cinnamon, tarragon, rosemary, thyme, cumin, and other favorite herbs and spices

Sweet potatoes, squash (including spaghetti), onions, and garlic

Olives, capers, roasted seaweed, popcorn, 70% dark chocolate, cacao powder

Protein powder, protein bars

Green tea, tea, coffee

Refrigerated Staples

Milk or alternative (almond milk, kefir, etc.), Kombucha, club soda or enhanced water

Greek yogurt; tempeh; parmesan, goat, feta, and/ or other cheese; organic butter; hummus; salsa

Salmon, chicken, turkey, eggs, lean meat

Greens, including spinach, kale, bok choy, romaine, cabbage (optional – buy pre-washed, chopped, and bagged)

Vegetables: avocado, cucumbers, broccoli, cauliflower, brussel sprouts, tomatoes, carrots, peppers, onions, beets, etc.

Fruit: blueberries, strawberries, raspberries, apples, grapes, cherries, kiwis, bananas, citrus, stone-fruits, melons, cranberries, etc.

Ginger, cilantro, basil, and other fresh herbs, roots

Freezer

Frozen berries for smoothies, edamame, frozen bananas (left overs), and fish/shrimp/meat for future use.

This list is not exhaustive; feel free to add and subtract according to your needs and preferences, as well as what is on your menu for the week.

Beyond Food

Now that you have made modifications in your home related to food and nutrition, it is time to step back and observe the environment you are living in. Do your surroundings invoke tranquility, comfort, pleasant memories, or the vibe you are wanting? Or is there clutter, noise, and disorganization?

What can you do or change to bring about the feeling that you want to have when you are in your home? You may want a unique feel in each room. A visualization exercise can help inspire ideas to help you transform your home into your idealized place.

As you imagine the following scenes, utilize all of your senses to capture the essence of that place or time and see if you can incorporate that into your current surroundings.

√ Where do you like to spend your leisure time?

√ Where were some of your favorite vacations?

√ What seasons are your favorite?

√ What colors appeal to you?

√ What are your favorite scents and sounds?

How can you bring aspects of the above into your home?

• Sound

  √ Music – Set the stage you want with the type of music you have playing, whether it is relaxing, inspiring, uplifting, or energizing.

  √ Water – Whether it is an indoor water fountain or an outdoor pond, not only is the sound of running water soothing, but it also generates negative ions which purify the air and promote a general sense of well-being.

• Scent

  √ Candles

  √ Potpourri on the stove (boil water on the stove with any mix of ingredients – cinnamon sticks, cloves, and vanilla evoke nurturing and comfort).

  √ You can utilize a diffuser for aromatherapy to bring in the scent of the mood you want to evoke.

    • Lemon – focused and calm
    • Pine – fresh and invigorating
    • Peppermint – energizing
    • Lavender – relaxing
    • Cinnamon – stimulating
    • Vanilla – nostalgic, contentment, comforting
    • Grapefruit – energizing
    • Tropical – memories of summer or vacation (pleasure)
    • Jasmine – earthy, calming, and uplifting
    • Bergamot – mood-lifting

- Sandalwood – woodsy, earthy, sensual

- Other _____

_____

- Color
  Think of the color palette that represents the scene that you want to duplicate:
  - Beige, white, and ocean blue evoke the seashore.
  - Fuchsia, orange-red, and yellow evoke the tropics.
  - Dark brown, turquoise, and silver evoke the southwest.
  - Navy, white, and yellow evoke lakeside and nautical.
  - Dark green, brown, and sky blue evoke forest and mountain.

  - Other _____

  _____

- Nature
  Bring nature in with plants, flowers, etc. Plants are natural air-purifiers and promote general well-being. Some of the easiest to grow include the spider plant, ficus/weeping fig, peace lily, Boston fern, snake plant, aloe vera, and bamboo palm.

Chapter 5 Recap

√ Be aware of environmental food cues.
  - Eat at the dining table, off of a plate, doing nothing else.
  - Do not eat in front of the TV or computer, or while reading.

√ Plan your meals and snacks.

√ Grocery shop from a list.

√ Keep healthy foods front and center

√ Don't bring high-risk food into the house.

Chapter 6 Summary

- What is Body-Image?
- Socio-Cultural Consciousness Raising
- Factors that Influence Body-Image Perception
  - Mood
  - Food Consumption
  - Comparisons
  - Developmental History: Puberty and Teasing
  - Family-of-Origin Influences
  - Negative Sexual Experiences and other Body Trauma
  - A Word on "Phantom Fat"
- Body-Image as a Concrete Representation of Self
  - Self-Image "Pie" Exercise
  - Body-Image "Pie" Exercise
- Letter to Your Body Exercise
- Body-Image as a Form of Communication
  - Weight as a Solution to Deeper Issues
  - Guided Imagery – "The Purpose Weight Serves"
- Body-Image "Real" versus "Ideal"
  - Body Satisfaction Graph
- Acceptance and Commitment Therapy and Cognitive Restructuring

HEALING BODY-IMAGE DISSATISFACTION

6

"You should clothe yourselves instead with the beauty that comes from within, the unfading beauty of a gentle and quiet spirit, which is so precious to God." – 1 Peter 3:4

Would you like to be able to appreciate your body where it's at? You can make peace with your body, even before you lose weight or change it in any way. When you are comfortable with your body, the less obsessed you will be with having to change it, aka "diet". Body-image satisfaction is your ticket out of the diet cycle.

An individual's body image is not an issue to be taken lightly. The conflict you have with your body goes beyond the superficial diagnosis of egocentricity or narcissism. How you view your body has a major impact on how you view yourself, how you think others see you, and your daily functioning. A preoccupation with appearance goes deeper than the outer image; it can affect the choices you make and goals you pursue. The consequences of having a poor body image can be significant – undermining self-confidence, promoting social isolation, inhibiting sexual expression, and it often precipitates chronic dieting that can lead to disordered eating.

Body-image has been defined as the mental image we form in our minds as a tridimensional unity involving physiological, psychological, and social factors. This image is the composite of perceptions, attitudes, and feelings towards one's body (Thompson, 1990). These concepts have been identified as two independent dimensions: body perception and body attitude (Raust-Von Wright, 1988).

Our body perception is how we actually see our physical appearance. Our body attitude encompasses a broad spectrum of feelings, beliefs, and emotional reactions towards the body and how we value it (Thompson, 1990 and Raust-Von Wright, 1988). There may be immense symbolism represented in your body-image.

Research shows that body-image dissatisfaction is independent of physical characteristics. Women of all shapes and sizes show a tendency to see themselves as overweight, even when they aren't (Cash, 1990). A healthy body-image means the mental picture of your body is accurate and the feelings, assessment, and relationship toward your body are positive (McManus, 2004).

In order to change this preoccupation with body-image, it is important to first understand some of the factors that create body-image dissatisfaction. Your body-image is formed out of every experience you have ever had: the manner in which your parents related to and touched (held or hit) your body, how your role-models valued their bodies, acceptance or rejection (teasing) you experienced from your peers, your developmental history, negative sexual experiences and other body trauma, and the way you perceive your body to fit or not fit cultural standards (Cash, 1990; Chernin, 1983; Orbach, 1979; Root, 1987; Thompson, 1990; Wooley and Lewis, 1989).

The body-image exercises I include focus on two different aspects of body-image: 1) healing the psychological issues that cloud how you perceive your body, and 2) how you can feel better about the body you actually have.

Socio-Cultural Consciousness Raising

There has been considerable research exploring the impact of culture and media/advertising on shaping body-image. The themes that have been addressed include: the influence of a patriarchal society, the social and economic inequality of women, the rejection of social norms and sex-role stereotyping, rebelling against external control, and feminine beauty as a metaphor for society's expectation of women (Chernin, 1983 and 1986; Freedman, 1986; Kilbourne, 1987; and Orbach, 1979 and 1982).

Ehrenreich and English (1978) noted that women have historically been willing to alter their bodies to match the current societal notion of beauty. Rodin and Striegel-Moore (1984) note that society reinforces the acceptance of women – and now men – altering their bodies to achieve beauty (foot binding, corsets, cosmetic surgery, etc.). Jill Kilbourne's pioneering *Still Killing Us Softly* video chronicled how body types go in and out of fashion. One only has to look at history to get a glimpse of the ideal of beauty for that era and what form the ideal woman was supposed to emulate. Body-image was a reflection of what society needed women to be at that time in history.

Jean Kilbourne's *Still Killing Us Softly* video series looks at the impact adverting has on women's body-image: how it has promoted distorted and destructive ideas of femininity, damaging gender stereotypes, and images that reinforce unrealistic and unhealthy perceptions of beauty, perfection, and sexuality. Women are objectified and sexualized. The fashion, entertainment, and media industries have bombarded women with role models for physical attractiveness that are unrealistic representations of real people.

> *"Slimness is marketed as beauty, success, love, sexuality, wealth, and happiness. Marketing has capitalized on trends by promoting self-consciousness and personal discontent, so that the consumer will often believe she needs the remedies the advertiser offers. The diet and fashion industries are making billions of dollars selling body-insecurity to women."* (Kilbourne, 1979)

Historically, external appearance has been a real source of women's social power. When a woman is struggling to find her place in society, it can be tempting to look outward (appearance) to define self. Since a woman's body is highly visible, it often becomes the arena in which she focuses her attention (Boskind-Lodahl, 1981; Chernin, 1983; and Orbach, 1979).

Men are not immune to being targeted by advertisers or the diet and fitness industries, although it is a relatively new phenomenon. Both women and men feel pressure to conform to today's image of attractiveness, and if they don't measure up, they may become self-critical. Consequently, dieting becomes the solution. Chronic dieting can lead to an obsession with food and disordered eating.

√ What can you do? Be a smart consumer. Be mindful of subliminal messages in advertising. You don't have to internalize the current cultural/media view of beauty.

√ Explore and challenge cultural/media influences. We must begin to question some of the ideas about weight and body-image that have been shaped by our current cultural climate.

√ In what ways do you feel culture and advertising has impacted your own body-image?

_____

_____

_____

_____

_____

_____

Body-Image Perception

Your body-image is the way you see and experience your body. It may not be the same as how you actually look or how others see you. How you perceive your body is greatly influenced not only by cultural factors, but psychological and physiological factors as well (Fairborn, 1985; Kaplan, 1980; Kearney-Cooke, 1988, Thompson, 1980).

Whenever you catch yourself assessing your body, there are certain things you can do to help see yourself more accurately. Always assess yourself in a **thinking** mode, not a **feeling** mode. How you feel you look and how you actually look are quite different (Thompson and Psaltis, 1988).

Factors that influence how you **feel** you look:

Mood

• When you are experiencing distressing emotions (depression, frustration, anxiety, etc.), you will likely have a negative perception of your world. This includes a negative perception of your body.

- If you are worried about an issue or disappointed in yourself, you may turn that focus onto your body instead of having to deal with the original problem. Your body/weight is concrete – you can see it. Conflicts are internal, abstract and often subconscious. This defense mechanism is called displacement. If you focus on your body and see it as okay, that would be the end of it and you would have to go back to thinking about the real issue. If you tell yourself you look overweight, you can obsess about that for hours, and the solution becomes a diet.

- There is a certain payoff for having a negative body-image; it helps you to defocus off the real issues. Negative feelings about your body may be symbolic of the dissatisfaction you have in other areas of your life.

What you can do:

   √ Be mindful of **not** looking in the mirror if you have had a difficult day or are in a negative mood.

   √ If you start thinking negatively about your body, ask yourself if there is something else that is bothering you.

   √ Journal or talk to someone about what is actually bothering you.

   √ Utilize healthy coping strategies to deal with negative emotions or disappointments in yourself.

Food Consumption

- Differentiate between feeling **full** and feeling **fat**. The sensation of being full increases the focus on your stomach. Your abdomen may be temporarily slightly distended during the digestion process; this is normal.

   √ Engage in a diversional activity after eating.

   √ Try eating six smaller meals a day, rather than three large ones.

Comparisons

- If you compare yourself with models or actresses (advertisements, media, etc.), what you see is often an illusion. You don't see the hours that are spent on make-up or hairstyle. Duct tape is often used to create cleavage, tape back thighs, and tape up buttocks. Make-up and spray-tan is used to contour face and body. Bodies are positioned to create a flattering pose and the camera captures the best angle. Photos are airbrushed and computer modified. These individuals may have personal trainers, chefs, and plastic surgeons. They may also have eating disorders. And yes, some are just born "beautiful" with great genetics.

What can you do?

√ Which messages from advertisers/media/culture (you need to be young, thin, sexy, glamorous, etc.) prevent you from accepting your body? _____

_____

_____

_____

√ If you don't "measure up," is it realistically in your grasp? There are different body types, body shapes, and different bone structures. Honor your own body's uniqueness. You are special just the way you are.

√ Remember, your reaction to your body-image is conditioned by culture. Now is the time to challenge these messages and change your views about your body that have been shaped by outside influences.

• If you compare yourself with friends, family members, or strangers (live representations, not on paper or other media), you may tend to maximize their positives and minimize their imperfections, while you do the opposite to yourself.

What can you do?

√ Don't just focus on the most attractive person in the room to compare yourself with. Look around the room and celebrate the diversity of beauty, body shapes, and sizes. There will always be someone more than or someone less than, in terms of physical appearance and the cultural norm at the time.

√ What do you think are your special physical attributes? _____

_____

_____

_____

√ Describe aspects of yourself that you have gotten positive feedback on: _____

_____

_____

_____

√ Remember, you have deeper qualities that can't be measured or compared, i.e., your character, your integrity, your spirituality, etc. What makes you unique? _____

_____

_____

Developmental History

These factors are relevant because their occurrence often increases the focus on your body (Wooley and Kearney-Cooke, 1987).

- **Puberty**
  This is a pivotal transitional time for both young men and women. Hormones are fluctuating, as are moods. Bodies are developing, changing, and growing. The normal biological change of additional adipose (fat) tissue for most adolescent girls can be quite distressing, as it is opposite of how the media is telling them to be (thin).

  Maturational timing has been shown to influence body-image. Girls who mature earlier than their peers often have a negative body-image, especially if they feel they are overweight, bigger busted, or taller than average. For men, the opposite seems to be true, as height and muscularity are valued (Thompson, 1990).

  √ How did your body maturation affect your body-image? _____

  _____

  _____

  _____

- **Teasing History**
  Adult men and women who were teased about their appearance as children have less satisfaction with their bodies as adults than those who were not teased. Being overweight in childhood causes an increase in teasing and a more negative body-image (Thompson, 1990).

  √ If you were you teased about your body or weight, how did it affect you? _____

  _____

  _____

  _____

  _____

  √ Did comments from a boyfriend or girlfriend affect your body-image? _____

  _____

  _____

  _____

√ Do you currently receive negative comments about your body from anyone and if so, how does it impact you? _____

_____

_____

_____

_____

How to Heal

√ Realize that today (in the present), the majority of people are not focusing on nor judging your body. It may feel like they are because it may be part of a core belief that you developed years ago. Adolescence is a developmental time period where many kids are looking, comparing, and judging. They were as insecure as you were (no matter whom they were). Unfortunately, an immature style of raising self-esteem is putting down someone else in order to lift yourself up. Thankfully, most people grow out of that and learn healthier ways to feel good about themselves *(see Diet Mentality chapter)*.

Family Influence

How your parents related to, commented on, touched, or didn't touch your body can impact how you relate to your body today. If you were not nurtured or were neglected in any way, that can impact how you care for your own body. Either or both parents may exhibit negative self-talk about their own body, or aim body/weight criticism at you directly or indirectly, by judging other people on their weight (Root, 1987).

Either or both parents may be overweight or have food or weight issues. They may be preoccupied with their own weight or shape and project this preoccupation onto obsessing about your weight and shape. If you grow up with this being the norm, you may come to believe that other people are focused on your weight. Again, this is typically not the case. Most people are caught up in their own lives, unless they have unresolved food and weight issues too.

Siblings and/or other members of the family may get caught up in food and weight issues as well. There may have been teasing or inappropriate comments, or there may have been a competitive atmosphere with weight/shape.

A mother may see her daughter as an extension and reflection of herself. If she is overinvested in her daughter, the daughter's attempt to separate and create an identity for herself may

168

manifest itself in dieting, especially if the mother is overweight (Kearney-Cooke, 1988). It may not actually be the mother's weight per se, but what it represents (mother's personality, role in the house or society, etc.). Another dynamic may be a thin mother trying to control her child's food intake, and the child/adolescents response is to "not be like mother" so they will rebel, sneak eat, and gain weight.

Puberty often marks a shift in a father's relationship with his daughter. The father may be uncomfortable with his daughter's changing body and may withdraw physical affection, make inappropriate comments, or cross boundaries (Maine, 2004).

√ How do you think your family influenced your body-image? _____

_____

_____

_____

_____

_____

What can you do?

√ Depending on the degree of dysfunction in your family-of origin, you may be able to challenge some of your core beliefs using cognitive restructuring. If you need the healing to go a little deeper, counseling or self-help books are good options.

√ Be mindful of family-of-origin patterns still occurring today. If you are still receiving critical comments about what you eat or your body/weight, maybe it's time to set some boundaries on the inappropriate remarks. You are an adult now and your family has no power over you unless you give it to them. If you find it difficult to assert yourself with your family, you may be caught in a re-enactment pattern – it feels as if you are still in the parent/young child dynamic, with no control and no voice. You are in the "freeze" mode of the "fight and flight" response and are experiencing "learned helplessness" (see Emotional Eating chapter). You may benefit from either self-help books on assertiveness or boundaries, or the support and guidance of counseling.

√ If you internalized messages from your family about your body, it is time to assess whether or not that information is even accurate. Cognitive restructuring and other body-image work can be helpful.

√ Utilize a strategy that I call your "Mental Shield." You can use this for self-esteem in general, body-image, or in any interpersonal situation where someone is being critical of you. Instead of being a "sponge" and absorbing the criticism, visualize your mental shield in front of you and the side that faces others has a mirror on it. So whatever anyone sends out reflects back on them, because it is really more about them. Even if there is a grain of truth in their feedback, if it is said in a demeaning way, it is really about their issues (their OCD, their narcissism, their insecurity, their need to control, etc.)

- *Example: You burn the toast. Your boyfriend says, "I can't believe you burnt the toast; you're so stupid." (The grain of truth is – you did burn the toast. Period. That doesn't mean you're stupid.) That comment is about him and his low self-esteem and need to control.*

Negative Sexual Experiences and other Body Trauma

√ Please see Emotional Eating chapter for in-depth discussion on this topic.

√ Use this space to journal your feelings and insights about how you feel your trauma

experience has impacted your body-image: _____

_____

_____

_____

_____

_____

_____

_____

_____

_____

_____

_____

A Word on "Phantom Fat"

Body-image distortion in Anorexia Nervosa is a commonly know phenomenon; even though the individual has lost a considerable amount of weight and may even be emaciated, they may still see their reflection in the mirror as overweight (Crisp and Kalucy, 1974). People who were formerly overweight often still carry that internal image with them. Cash (2008) labels this occurrence "phantom fat," which references the "phantom limb" experience that amputees often feel after losing part of their body. Most researchers feel that the image in the brain hasn't caught up to the new smaller body, especially for individuals who were obese for many years or experienced being overweight in childhood. This is a temporary state for most individuals.

√ Retrain your brain using cognitive restructuring techniques.

√ Use perceptual feedback procedures to help see yourself more accurately: before and after photographs, videotape, outlining shape.

√ Reattribution training (how you feel you look vs. how you actually look)
  Use the analogy of someone who is color blind learning to utilize a stop light, not by color but by which bulb lights up.
  - Keep an outfit in your original size and try it on once a month.
  - Compare the current number on the scale with the number you originally weighed. Keep a monthly graph.
  - Compare your current clothing size with the size you wore at your highest weight. Keep a monthly graph.

Body-Image as a Concrete Representation of Self

We looked at the role family-of-origin and childhood events have in shaping how you see yourself and developing some of the traits you have. If you have not formed a strong self-identity or your self-worth is based on external validation (approval from others or conforming to media standards), you may be trying to solve your identity and esteem problems by focusing on your body, a concrete, visible representation of self (Inhelder and Piaget, 1958).

Believing that altering your shape will bring you self-confidence and happiness, you begin your next diet. Resisting the natural urge to eat gives you a sense of control and personal accomplishment (Bruch, 1978, Orbach, 1979 and Chernin, 1981). The attention you receive from the weight-loss acts as a reinforcement and validation that "weight matters."

Your body-image is an aspect of your self-image, but when you overvalue it in regard to determining your self-worth, you may end up spending an inordinate amount of time and energy obsessing about food and weight instead of developing your confidence and abilities in other areas.

When your self-identity is solid and based on your intrinsic worth and who you believe you are, incoming negativity does not shake your self-confidence. This is the difference between internal validation (looking within for approval) and external validation (needing someone else to think you're okay). Healthy self-esteem motivates and empowers. When you value yourself, you are able to communicate assertively because you believe your feelings and needs have value. When you feel good about who you are, you are able to treat others well and expect the same in return.

When you feel you have intrinsic worth (as you are), you are more inclined to take care of yourself and your body. This includes basic hygiene; eating healthful foods; giving your body movement, relaxation, and adequate sleep; and not engaging in harmful behaviors.

Body-image, especially for women, is closely tied to self-concept. A negative body-image often causes a decline in self-esteem (Cash, 1990 and Thompson, 1980). Conversely, low self-esteem will influence how you perceive your body-image.

There are a number of approaches to feeling better about yourself. Your internal dialogue offers a starting point to help you determine the areas you need to modify. Cognitive restructuring has been the gold standard used to modify negative self-talk (Mckay and Fanning, 1987). Challenging and changing core beliefs may require healing past issues *(see Emotional Eating and Diet Mentality chapters).*

Neff (2011) suggests that building self-compassion is a healthier way to promote emotional well-being. She defines self-compassion as 1) changing your critical, judgmental self-talk to being understanding and supportive; 2) framing your personal experience in light of a shared human experience; and 3) awareness of things as they truly are (not exaggerating a situation or engaging in unhealthy self-pity).

You don't have to be perfect; be "authentic" (Epstein, 2015). Be the best expression of yourself that you can be. If you have a bad day – give yourself a hug, apologize if you need to, offer grace and forgiveness if it's on them, show compassion to self and others – and then move on.

You are not your body. Your body-image is only one aspect of your self-image. When you learn to define and value yourself for your inner qualities, you will begin to be less obsessed about your external appearance.

Self-Image "Pie" Exercise:

How much of your self-image "pie" does body-image currently occupy? How would you like it to be? (Fairburn, 1985)

Example

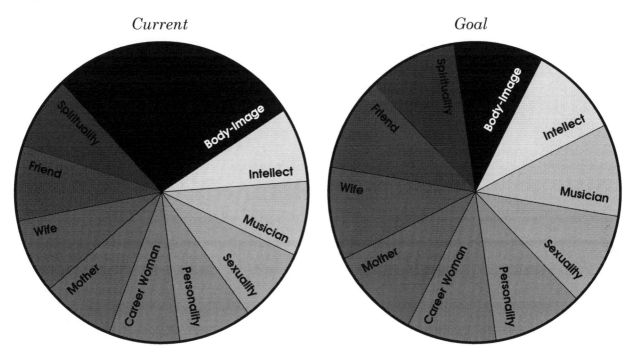

Current

Goal

Your Circles

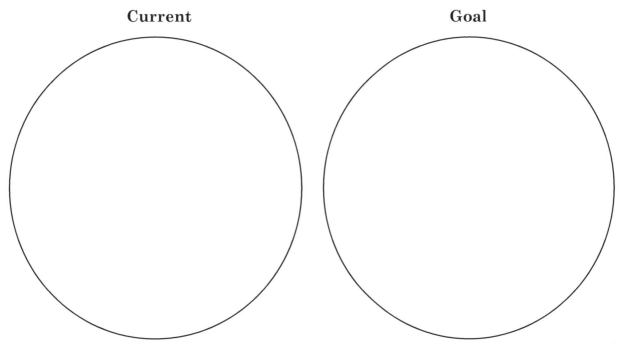

Current

Goal

What are other aspects of who you are that are worthwhile?

- Interpersonal (roles, relationships)
- Intellect
- Spirituality
- Sexuality
- Career, community involvement
- Other _____
- List your assets, qualities and gifts:

  - What makes you special/unique: _____

    _____

    _____

  - Your character/integrity: _____

    _____

    _____

  - What you value: _____

    _____

    _____

  - Your purpose in life: _____

    _____

    _____

  - Your personality: _____

    _____

    _____

  - Your abilities/skills: _____

    _____

_____

_____

- Your achievements: _____

_____

_____

- Your interests and hobbies: _____

_____

_____

- Your dreams, aspirations, and goals: _____

_____

_____

Limitations:

- (I would like myself better if I were less...) _____

_____

_____

- (I would like myself better if I were more...) _____

_____

_____

√ What can I do to overcome these limitations? _____

_____

_____

It may seem like it is easier to control/change concrete, tangible things like food and weight versus the abstract – personality, character, roles, relationships, etc. This pattern may have started in childhood or early adolescence when your thinking style was concrete (normal developmental stage). Although you have advanced to abstract thinking in many areas, if you experienced any childhood trauma, there may be areas where your development may have been arrested; you may still think or respond in the manner that you would have at that earlier age. Disordered eating and obsessing about body weight and size are two examples of concrete, regressive coping styles. (They "make sense" at that earlier age, but interfere with functioning now.)

Body-Image Pie

Your body-image is more than just your physical appearance (beauty object). This exercise will guide you to view your body for all of its capacities.

- Expand how you define your appearance (twinkle in your eyes, your laugh, your energy level, how you "carry yourself").

- When you walk into a room, people notice your self-confidence more than they notice your appearance.

    She is clothed with strength and dignity and she laughs without fear of the future. Proverbs 31:25

- Appreciate the other roles your body provides: autonomy, intimacy, communication, sensory, athletic, artistic, sensual/sexual, reproductive, spiritual, etc.

    "Don't you know that your body is the temple of the Holy Spirit, who lives in you and was given to you by God?" 1 Corinthians 6:19

- To help increase your awareness of the functions your body is capable of, imagine if you didn't have legs. Instead of, "my thighs are fat," you would appreciate being able to have legs to walk on the beach or run around with your children. Instead of, "my arms are flabby," you would appreciate being able to wave to your neighbor, rock your baby, or hug your friend.

- The majority of ways you use or depend on your body are independent of your weight and shape. Granted, your health matters and may impact how your body functions in certain roles. But your grandchild doesn't care if Grandma is "fluffy." You don't have to have a perfect figure to do yoga. You can be in a loving relationship no matter what the number on the scale says.

- How much of your body-image pie do you give to appearance?

Example

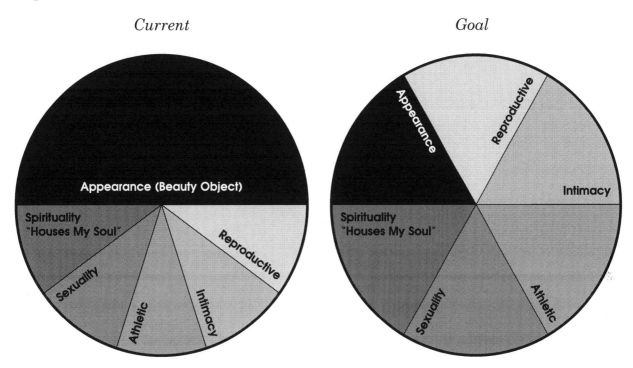

Current · Goal

Your Circles

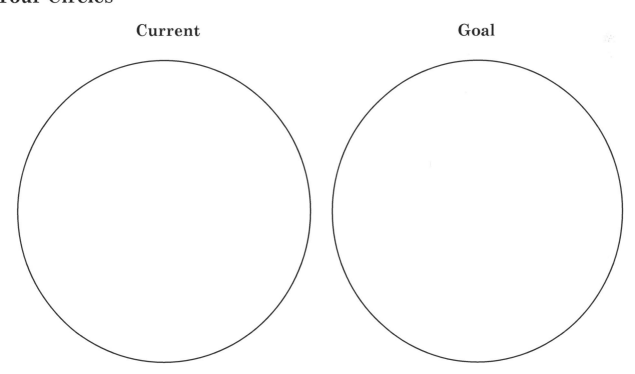

Current · Goal

Letter Writing Exercise

There is no right or wrong way to approach this exercise. It is comprised of two parts. First, allow your "body" to write a letter to you. Next, write a letter to your body.

Some people find that when they allow their body to talk, they will get insights into how their body is being treated, what their body has experienced and still carries around, etc. They may begin to experience more compassion towards their body, so when they write back, they are kinder and less critical.

Dear _____(your name)

_____

_____

_____

_____

_____

_____

_____

_____

_____

_____

_____

_____

_____

_____

Dear Body,

_____

_____

_____

_____

_____

_____

_____

_____

_____

_____

_____

_____

_____

_____

_____

_____

_____

_____

_____

_____

_____

_____

_____

_____

Body-Image (and Disordered Eating) as a Form of Communication

An entire chapter of this workbook covers emotional eating, discussing how food is used to deal with or avoid feelings and issues. Food can also be used to symbolically communicate feelings (Crisp, 1981 and Roth, 1983). Refusing to eat may convey self-punishment – "I don't deserve to eat," assert autonomy – "You can't control what I eat," or anger (passive-aggressive) – "You want me to eat, so I won't."

Overeating may be a way to "stuff" anger, assert autonomy, or balance a quid pro quo, i.e., "If you're going to drink/gamble/smoke, I am going to eat." These are only a few of the examples of how eating/not eating can be used to communicate indirectly in interpersonal relationships. This often happens when the individual is coping in a concrete regressive style (Levine, 1985 and Sperley, 1987) and is either lacking in self-esteem or communication skills (assertiveness, conflict resolution) and/or they are too afraid to use their voice i.e., shy, passive, anxious, or "re-enacting" old patterns (Boskind-Lodahl, 1981; Chernin, 1983 and 1986; Kaplan, 1980; Orbach, 1979 and 1982; and Wooley and Lewis, 1989).

√ Are you aware of how you may be using food/eating to communicate?_____

_____

_____

_____

_____

_____

√ How can you express yourself and get your needs met without using food to

communicate for you? _____

_____

_____

_____

_____

_____

_____

Weight as a Solution to Deeper Issues

Now that you have the insight of how you may be using food to symbolically communicate, it's time to look at how you may be using your body/weight to communicate. Your body has always been a way to express yourself, from the clothes you wear, to the way you walk, to the way you use non-verbal communication (eye contact, posture, hand gestures, etc.).

The internal conflicts that you may be experiencing may be too abstract to be expressed verbally, or you may feel that you do not have a voice (passivity, anxiety, or fear), (Chernin, 1983). As discussed earlier in the workbook, having a trauma history is common with disordered eating. Trauma can happen at an age when you don't have the words to describe how you are feeling, but your body records the memory, therefore re-enactment may occur via the body (Van Der Kolk, 2014).

√ What does being "thin" mean to you? _____

_____

_____

_____

√ "If I were thin, women would…" _____

_____

_____

_____

√ "If I were thin, men would…" _____

_____

_____

_____

√ What does being overweight mean to you? _____

_____

_____

_____

√ "If I am overweight, women will..." _____

_____

_____

_____

√ "If I am overweight, men will..." _____

_____

_____

_____

√ How do you use your body to communicate? _____

_____

_____

_____

_____

√ What does your extra weight do for you? _____

_____

_____

_____

_____

Examples

Thin may communicate or mean:

- Power
- Control
- Popularity
- Sexuality
- Independence

- Might threaten friendships
- Might have the self-esteem to leave marriage
- The opposite sex will be attracted to me

- _____

_____

_____

Very underweight may communicate or mean:

- Need help
- Need someone to take care of me
- Fear of sexuality

- _____

_____

_____

Extra weight may communicate or mean:

- Protection
- Safety
- Boundaries
- Power
- "My right to take up space"
- "I can blame weight for failing or not achieving something."
- "I am not a threat to the same sex."
- Fear of intimacy
- Maternal or paternal image.
- May play a role in marital dynamics, i.e., punishment for spouse's infidelity.

- _____

√ How else can you communicate these feelings, needs, or issues? _____

_____

_____

_____

Visualization Exercise: Gaining Insight into the Purpose of Your Weight

Guided imagery is a useful strategy to go beyond intellectualization and tap into emotion and body language. It may provide a deeper understanding of the role weight serves in your life or relationships. It may be easier to "release" the weight once you gain insight and deal with or heal the underlying issue (Hutchinson, 1985; Kearney-Cooke, 1988; Root, 1987; Wooley and Kearney-Cooke, 1987). (If you have a trauma history, or this exercise triggers uncomfortable feelings, memories, or thoughts of self-harm, please seek professional support.)

- Get into a relaxed position in a reasonably quiet environment.

- Take slow, deep, relaxing breaths.

- You have control over this guided imagery. You can stop at any time and return to relaxed breathing and visualizing a safe, relaxing scene. You can break this exercise up into two or three focal points.

- Visualize yourself at your lightest, healthiest weight (before your first significant weight gain). How do you feel in your body? Notice what your wearing, your hairstyle, any cosmetics or jewelry that you may have on. In your mind's eye, look at yourself, your body, in a full length mirror. What do you notice? How old are you? What messages are you hearing about your body?

- Now move ahead to when you started gaining weight. Was it gradual? Did it occur after any certain time in your development or any specific event? Visualize your body adding on each layer (stage) of weight gain.

- Visualize yourself at your highest weight. In your mind's eye, look at yourself in a full length mirror. What do you see? How do you feel in your body? What messages are you hearing about your body?

- Visualize yourself at this weight in a public setting. How are you feeling? What thoughts or images are coming up for you?

- Visualize yourself around family, current or family-of-origin. What feelings or thoughts are coming up for you?

- Return to focusing on your breathing, slow deep breaths.

- Now visualize yourself letting go of the weight. You are at your ideal weight. In your mind's eye, look at yourself in a full length mirror. What do you see? How do you feel in your body?

- Visualize yourself at this weight in a public setting. Walking down a street. How are you feeling? What thoughts or images are coming up for you? Do you need your extra weight for anything?

- Visualize yourself at your ideal weight around family, current or family-of origin. What feelings or thoughts are coming up for you?

- Return to focusing on your breathing, slow deep breaths.

- Visualize yourself where you are at now.

Use this time to journal any thoughts, feelings, or new insights that may have come up for you. What is your body-image story? (Seigel, 2015)

_____

_____

_____

_____

_____

_____

_____

_____

_____

_____

_____

the *glow approach*

How can you rewrite this story?

_____

_____

_____

_____

_____

_____

_____

_____

_____

_____

_____

_____

_____

_____

_____

_____

_____

_____

_____

_____

_____

_____

_____

_____

Body-Image: Ideal vs. Real

The further your ideal body-image is from your real (actual) shape, the greater your body-image dissatisfaction will be. Many of the body-image exercises you have been working on have addressed your psychological body-image and the factors that influence how you feel about your body, which create distortions in how you see your body.

When you begin to have compassion for your body, and when you begin to appreciate all that your body is and does, you will likely be able to see your actual body more realistically. That should help close the gap a bit (distance between ideal and real).

The next step is to realistically view your body: body type, shape, bone structure, muscularity, etc. These are the genetics you are born with. It is also important to look at where you're at in terms of the aging process. Like it or not, menopause does impact how and where weight is gained (see Physiology chapter). Your weight history and set point can also influence what amount of weight loss is manageable long-term. Taking these factors into consideration should help you have more realistic expectations about what an attainable "ideal" is. Let your own body be your guide.

Learning to appreciate your body for what it is and what it can do, and accepting your body as it is, doesn't mean you can't do anything to modify it. Healthy eating and non-compulsive exercise are appropriate ways to reduce weight (if needed).

Exercise is the best way to tone and modify your body shape; you will lose intramuscular and subcutaneous adipose tissue (fat). As the intramuscular fat is lost, total muscle mass will increase and a small weight gain may occur. Although muscle weighs more than fat, it also takes up less space than fat, so you will lose inches and see a decrease in clothing size. (This is a good reminder to not just focus on the number on the scale to determine your progress.) Intramuscular fat loss changes your body's shape. Firmness and toning are the result of exercise, not diet.

Research shows that any type of exercise increases body-image satisfaction, because you are focusing on what your body can do. Activity that incorporates mind-body movements such as yoga, tai chi, walking meditation, etc. facilitates integration and a deeper connection to your body.

Strive to focus on and emphasize your assets. Take the focus off and de-emphasize your perceived imperfections. You can do this by clothing style, color, and type; as well as utilizing accessories and cosmetics.

Body Satisfaction Graph

Individuals who are more dissatisfied with their body tend to break it into parts and compare that part with what they feel is ideal. Part of promoting body-image satisfaction is integrating these body parts into a whole body/whole person. In this exercise we will first utilize a graph to begin where you're at now in how you perceive your body (Slade, Dewey, Newton, Browdie, and Kiemle, 1989).

Rate your satisfaction with the following parts of your body. Place a check in the column that best describes your satisfaction with each body part. Write what you like about each part and what you would like to change.

	Very Satisfied	Generally Satisfied	Indifferent or Neutral	Somewhat Dissatisfied	Very Dissatisfied
Hair					
Face					
Shoulders					
Arms					
Hands					
Breasts/Chest					
Waist					
Abdomen/ Stomach					
Hips/Buttocks					
Thighs					
Lower Legs					
Calves					
Feet					
Your Body					

The goals of this exercise are:

1) To gradually improve upon how you label your body. If you are mostly in the far right hand columns (dissatisfaction), then your first move is to begin to use neutral terminology to describe that body part. You can use information from the exercises that you completed earlier. (Non-judgment)

- Example: Thighs – If you put a check in the "dissatisfied" column and wrote, "I want them to be smaller and less flabby." You could change that to a more neutral statement, i.e., "my legs are strong and they allow me to exercise."

2) Next, we want to look at what your ideal body-image is or what that body part would look like to meet your ideal image.

- Example: "My ideal stomach would be flat, concave, and muscular.

3) Next, try to be as realistic as you can be with describing what your body part/shape actually looks like. (Acceptance)

- Example: "My shape is more endomorph/mesomorph (curvy and muscular), so the shape would never be flat

4) Next, try to modify your "ideal" to make it more attainable.

- *Example: "My stomach shape will never be flat, but it could be more toned."*

5) What can you do to realistically change this body part (in a healthy manner)?

- *Example: "I can eat a healthy diet. I can do a moderate amount of cardio, strength training, and abdominal work."*

6) How can you use clothes or accessories to modify your shape or body part?

- *Example: "I can accentuate a different body part to highlight my assets and draw the focus away from my perceived flaw."*

Remember:

√ The closer your actual shape is to your ideal (hoped for) shape, the less body dissatisfaction you will have.

√ Do not characterize your whole appearance based on a single feature.

√ Focus on a body part that does please you.

√ You are the sum of all of your parts. Start to look at your body/yourself as a whole person.

"You should clothe yourselves instead with the beauty that comes from within, the unfading beauty of a gentle and quiet spirit, which is so precious to God." – 1 Peter 3:4

Acceptance and Commitment Therapy (ACT) is a promising approach to use with chronic body-image dissatisfaction. ACT helps the client identify what they value in life and determine whether or not their behaviors are helping them move in these valued life directions (Hayes, 1999; Kroll, 2017). Clients are taught to gain distance from thoughts and recognize that thoughts are simply a form of internal experiences, not necessarily a truth. For example, "I am having a thought that my stomach is too big," rather than simply, "My stomach is too big."

√ What does your negative body-image keep you from doing, and are you ready to face your fear and do it anyway? What is the worst thing that could happen?

_____

_____

_____

_____

_____

_____

_____

_____

√ Be mindful of your self-talk and remember to substitute – "This is just a thought…"

Cognitive Restructuring is also a useful tool in challenging negative self-talk about your body, weight, or the scale (Agras, 1987; Meichenbaum, 1985; and Root, 1987) *(see Diet Mentality chapter).*

The best beauty product is to have a life. A real life. With challenges, disappointments, stress, and laughter. The much-touted inner beauty is a natural radiance that comes as a result of mental and emotional involvement. The increased blood demand for oxygen of a busy brain attracts blood to the head, resulting in the luminous bloom on your forehead and cheeks. Your complexion glows, your eyes shine…[sic] – Veronique Vienne, *from The Art of Imperfection.*

Chapter 6 Recap

√ You can transform your body-image and learn to appreciate the body you were born with.

√ Utilize self-compassion towards your body, as you gain greater understanding of your history and the impact it has on your body-image.

√ Don't let the number on the scale define you.

√ Don't look in the mirror when you're having a bad day; it won't be an accurate reflection of who you really are. Spend less time in front of mirrors in general.

√ Realize that your body-image is only one aspect of your self-image. Learn to define yourself from within.

√ Appreciate your body for all of its capacities, not just for its relevance as a beauty object.

√ Focus on a part of your body that does please you and/or look at your body as a whole.

√ Accept the reality that bodies come in a variety of shapes and sizes. Be realistic in your expectations that you have for your body.

√ You get to decide what body size fits you; let your own body be your guide.

√ Learn to use your voice so your body-image doesn't need to communicate for you.

√ You can let go of the weight as you come to understand the purpose it serves.

√ Do things for yourself that are special right now, instead of waiting until you "lose weight."

√ Don't avoid activities that you enjoy, even if they call attention to your weight or shape. Remind yourself that you deserve to do things that you enjoy.

√ Engage in physical activity for the joy of feeling your body move.

√ Beauty transcends physical features. When you have peace with who you are on the inside, it radiates on the outside. Your inner glow creates that outer glow. That is what makes you beautiful!

Chapter 7 Summary

- Transformation is About Change
  - In relationship with food
  - In role of food
  - In "diet" mentality
  - In lifestyle choices
- Coping with Life without Using Food
- Balance Strategies for Weight-Loss and Weight Maintenance
  - Tier approach
  - Planning and Compensating
  - Get Rid of "Cheat" Day – Replace with Balance Strategies
  - Plan B
- Reset (Getting Back on Track)
- Understanding and Preventing Slips and Relapse
- Recovering from an Over-Eating Episode
- Managing Your Food/Weight Issues
- Strategies for Successful Weight-Loss Maintenance

SUSTAINABLE MAINTENANCE

7

"God grant me the serenity to accept the things that I cannot change; courage to change the things that I can; and wisdom to know the difference." - Reinhold Neibuhr

**Create Balance in Your Life and How You Nourish Your
body • mind • soul • spirit**

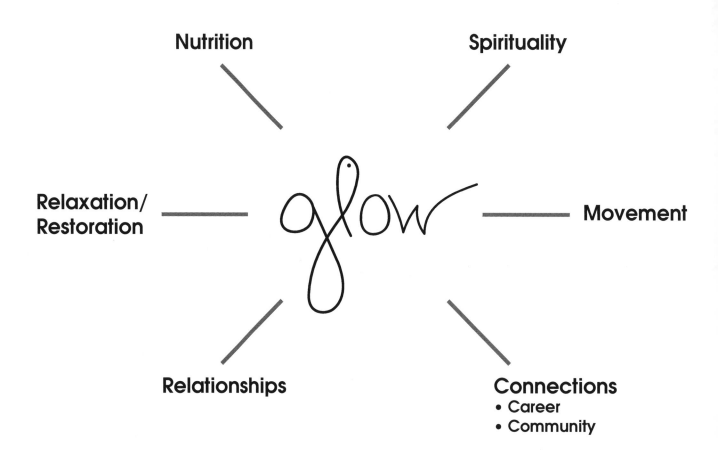

Nutrition

Spirituality

Relaxation/
Restoration

Movement

Relationships

Connections
• Career
• Community

glow approach versus "diet mentality"

"diet mentality"	glow approach
Willpower ➔	Eating with Awareness
Something you go on and off ➔	Lifestyle Changes
Deprivation ➔	Balance
Can't have ➔	What does your body need?
On or Off diet (all/none) ➔	Plan and Compensate
Good/Bad food ➔	Food will not define your self-worth: Eat without shame or guilt
Exercise connected to dieting ➔	Exercise is a part of lifestyle and connected to something else, like stress reduction, mood enhancement, etc.
Rigid food plan ➔	Tier approach with food. Weight-loss plan should look very close to weight maintenance plan
Food is friend/enemy ➔	Healthy relationship with food

**Change your relationship with food –
Transform your life .. Get the *glow*!**

A weight-loss plan only works if you stay with it, so the plan you choose needs to fit **you** (your preferences, personality, and your lifestyle). Your weight-loss plan should look fairly close to your maintenance plan in terms of nutritional choices and lifestyle changes to help insure a smooth transition versus going "off the diet" and back to old patterns. The goal is to find balance in your food choices and lifestyle.

Traditionally, a "diet" was something that had an endpoint. Unfortunately, this is also the point where most "dieters" return to their former eating patterns. This "all or none style" is common with emotional/compulsive eaters, especially if the "diet" was restrictive and induced a feeling of deprivation.

You will be more successful with your weight loss and maintenance when the changes you make are gradual and realistic. There should not be a sense of deprivation, but of balance and moderation. No one is telling you what to eat. It's you listening to your body. Put the focus on nourishing your body, your health, and how food makes your mind and body feel. Discover a way of eating that you enjoy, balances your nutritional needs, satisfies your hunger, and helps you reach your goals.

Transform Your Life

Transformation is about change: change in your relationship with food, change in the role of food, change in your diet mentality, and change in lifestyle.

Change

- In Relationship with Food
- In Role of food – Nutrition
- In "Diet" Mentality
- In Lifestyle Choices

Change in Relationship with Food

Have you learned to differentiate between physical hunger and emotional hunger or other non-hunger food cues?

_____

_____

_____

Have you been able to identify the roles that food or weight has served in your life?

_____

_____

_____

_____

_____

Have you been able to find alternative ways of coping that will fill the void if you let go of the emotional eating?

_____

_____

_____

_____

_____

- Gain insight into the purpose(s) of symptoms and the price you pay.
  Most people are able to let go of the emotional eating/weight when they are tired of the negative consequences **and** have found adequate substitutes for the role food/weight has played. When food/weight no longer serves a purpose, the price you pay outweighs any benefits of holding on to the symptoms.

  - Purpose of symptoms (pros) _____

    _____

    _____

    _____

    _____

    _____

    _____

Price you pay (cons) _____

_____

_____

_____

_____

_____

_____

Change in the Role of Food: Nutrition

• Change in mindset: from "diet" focus to health focus. No one is telling you what to eat.

It's you listening to your body. How does the food make your body feel? How is this food hurting, helping, or healing your body?

Have you learned what foods "work" for you and what your mind/body needs? _____

_____

_____

_____

_____

Have you learned which foods "work" for you for weight-loss? _____

_____

_____

_____

_____

Have you learned what foods don't work for you and cause symptoms? _____

_____

_____

Change in "Diet" Mentality:

- Have you made the change in mindset from "dieting" to lifestyle changes? _____

  _____

  _____

  _____

- Have you decreased or stopped the all/none, good/bad, restrict/binge patterns and replaced them with the concept of **balance** by using the "Tier Approach" and "planning and compensating?"_____

  _____

  _____

  _____

Change in Lifestyle:

- Have you been able to identify the areas in your life where there was a void? _____

  _____

  _____

  _____

- Have you created balance in your life in the areas of work/play, recreation/rest, and physical activity/relaxation strategies?

  Work: _____

  _____

  _____

  Play/Recreation: _____

  _____

  _____

Rest: _____

_____

_____

_____

Physical Activity/Movement: _____

_____

_____

Relaxation Strategies:_____

_____

_____

_____

Are you "full" filled? _____

_____

_____

_____

Are you involved in healthy, fulfilling relationships? _____

_____

_____

_____

Do you feel a connection to others/and your community?_____

_____

_____

_____

Do you have a purpose, passion, and/or spirituality that brings meaning to your life?

_____

_____

_____

Transformation Is Also About Choice:

Taking personal responsibility for your life and not helping to create "lifestyle" diseases.

- **Choice**
    - In what you put into your body. Take charge of your health destiny!
    - In how you cope with life issues.

Individuals who succeed at maintaining their weight loss have learned how to cope with life issues without using food. They have let go of "learned helplessness" and feel empowered to be in control of their food choices.

Granted, if life hands you major challenges or stressors, it is challenging to "diet" at the same time. A "diet" is one more thing to try to manage. However, instead of allowing the challenge or stressor to become an excuse to fall back into old eating habits, you can choose to use the Plan B strategy. *(See page 203 and Appendix H.)*

Do you believe that you have the ability to make lasting changes? What do you need to do to mobilize internal strengths and external resources to help you feel empowered and motivated?

_____

_____

_____

_____

_____

_____

Successful maintainers keep their focus on the big picture — **why** it is important to them to eat healthy or lose weight, versus the momentary instant gratification of food.

You are confronted by food choices every day, so you need to remind yourself every morning what your motivation is for healthy eating and/or losing weight. **What is your motivation?**

_____

_____

_____

_____

_____

_____

_____

Regaining Lost Weight

Why do you think you regain the weight you lose? _____

_____

_____

_____

_____

_____

_____

Do you identify with any of the commonly cited reasons?

- "Diet" is restrictive, so when the diet ends, you fall back into former eating patterns (all or none).

- You start "testing" the effects of reintroducing favorite foods and gradually fall back into former patterns.

- You pair exercise with "dieting," and once the "diet" is over, you stop exercising.

- You stop doing everything you were doing to get the weight off instead of making lifestyle changes.

- You fall back into emotional eating, "diet" mentality, and ignore environmental food cue exposure (eating in front of the TV, etc.).

- You get nervous when others start to notice and comment on your weight loss, triggering unresolved body-image issues *(see Body-image chapter).*

- Other _____

Balance Strategies for Weight-Loss and Weight-Loss Maintenance:

- **Tier Approach** *(See Diet Mentality chapter.)*

- **Planning and Compensating** *(See Diet Mentality chapter.)*

- **Getting Rid of "Cheat" Day: Replace with Balance Strategies**

The very definition of cheat invokes the feeling of doing something wrong or bad. Glow encourages letting go of negativity – "bad" food, "sneak" eating, "cheat" day. Typically, for most emotional eaters, "cheat" day triggers all/none thinking and behaviors. It keeps people in their old behavioral patterns instead of practicing new habits.

If you need a break from your Plan A (Optimal food plan), take a day and focus on maintenance (tier 3), and use planning and compensating to balance calories. Even if you go over a bit, you can still compensate for calories the following day, or plan for some extra activity.

- **Plan B**
  - Useful as a transition after a vacation, holiday, etc.
  - An option if "too busy" or "too stressed"

The reality of "dieting," and even just eating more healthful, does require time and energy. Some days, weeks, or months, because of circumstances, you may not have the time or energy to follow your "optimal plan." Enter Plan B: quicker, easier options that are alternatives to falling back into less healthy patterns. There is no one Plan B. It is yours to design. *(See Appendix H.)*

It is helpful to have options for all three meals and snacks written down, so you don't have to think about creating a list during that difficult time. *(See Appendix H for simple meal ideas.)*

Plan B Ideas:

Breakfast

- Pre-made protein shakes
- Protein bars

- Instant steel-cut oatmeal
- Banana with peanut butter

- Eggs
- Whole-grain toast with peanut butter or avocado
- Yogurt with chopped nuts
- Buy pre-cut fruit to add to meal (optional)

- Add your ideas: _____

_____

_____

_____

_____

Lunch

- Cheese sticks wrapped with sliced meat
- Tuna pack and canned 3-bean salad or avocado half
- Canned soup (healthy option)

- Frozen dinner (healthy option)

- Prepared salad mix, add rotisserie chicken

- Pre-cut vegetables and hummus

- Drive-thru: salad or cheese burger and apple slices
- Prepared sushi

- Add your ideas: _____

_____

_____

_____

Dinner

- Pick up precooked chicken (shredded or rotisserie) and serve with either a sweet potato (microwave) or brown rice (90 seconds in the microwave) and canned green beans.

- Use the grill or Crockpot to cook meat or poultry, root vegetables, etc.

- Utilize pre-cut fresh, canned, or frozen vegetables.
- Canned salmon – mix with quick brown rice and steamed vegetables for a "bowl."
- Buy pre-cut vegetables in a steamer bag for quick cooking in the microwave or stir-fry with a bottled sauce; add chopped cashews to the stir-fry.
- Microwave spaghetti squash; serve with marinara and parmesan cheese.
- Thaw frozen shrimp – chop and mix with sliced avocado and salsa for a quick shrimp ceviche.

- _____

  _____

Snacks

- Yogurt
- 1 oz. dark chocolate
- Pre-made (healthy) popcorn
- Hummus and baby carrots
- Fresh fruit and fresh vegetables
- Hard-boiled eggs

- _____

  _____

Reset (Getting back on track after a vacation, holiday, relapse, or weight gain)

- Plan
- Schedule
- Structure

  √ Yep, it's time to utilize your awareness record, food/mood diary, nutrition app, daily planner, etc. (whatever you use to record, schedule, or make lists).

  √ Determine if you are willing and able to return to your Plan A (your optimal food plan). If not, this is where Plan B fits in.

  √ Start with a meal plan for the week, and then make your grocery list. Use your day planner to schedule in times to exercise.

√ Monitor your awareness record for triggers. Self-monitoring is a must if you have had multiple slips, a relapse, or unaccounted weight gain.

Understanding and Preventing Relapse

Relapse prevention is a cognitive-behavioral approach with the goal of identifying and preventing high-risk situations for relapse. You will use coping skills and self-control strategies, and develop a greater sense of mastery. You will learn to utilize your strengths and begin to change patterns that are no longer effective.

- When individuals attempt to change a behavior, setbacks (slips) are highly probable.

- How you define or handle the slip determines the outcome. It is important to understand the difference between a slip (lapse) and a relapse.

- A lapse (slip) is one violation of a self-imposed rule, whereas a relapse is a string of slips that lead to the previous problematic behavior pattern.

- How you respond to the slip will determine whether or not it triggers a relapse or moves you in the direction of a more solid recovery.

- Slips are part of recovery.

- Slips are an opportunity for self-growth, to learn what your high-risk areas are, so you can be prepared for the next time that you are in that situation.

- Slips are more commonly associated with situational factors, whereas relapses typically occur during negative emotional states and stressful events.

- Negative moods may increase the chance that a slip will progress into a relapse.

Preventing Slips: Be Aware of Your Triggers

Increase your awareness of your high-risk situations. If you have a slip, assess these areas for the possible trigger(s):

- Emotions
  - Internal: angry, anxious, sad, depressed, lonely, bored, stressed, etc.
  - Interpersonal: conflicts, relationship issues, work pressures, lifestyle or value conflicts, acute or chronic problems, etc.
  - Unresolved trauma or loss
  - Other _____

- Cognitions (thoughts)

- Distorted beliefs about food, weight, body, slips, etc.
- Distorted beliefs about self, others, situations, etc.
- Other _____

- Environmental
  - Conditioned Eating: food cues
  - Social situations: holidays, vacations, celebrations, restaurant eating, entertaining, parties, etc.
  - Other _____

- Physical State
  - Internal: hungry (intake too low or waiting too long between meals, or not enough protein or healthy fat), tired, thirsty, hormonal, medication side-effects, etc.
  - High-risk foods for overeating: _____
  - Other _____

Recovering from an Over-Eating Episode

You may feel disorganized after overeating or bingeing. Have this guide readily available to use as a step-by-step plan, to prevent falling back into your habitual response pattern (restricting, purging, negative self-talk, etc.).

1) Go to a room away from the kitchen or bathroom.

2) Monitor your thoughts for negativity or cognitive distortions.
   - Be mindful of how you talk to yourself after a slip. Be careful not to see the slip as a sign of personal weakness or failure, but instead, attribute the slip to the external precipitating factors (things you can change).

3) Challenge the irrational thoughts with cognitive restructuring.
   - Use compassionate self-talk.

4) Get involved in an alternative activity for distraction.

5) Try to resume normal eating at the next meal. Use balance strategies.

6) Determine the factors that contributed to the slip (see above for list of triggers).
   - What were you feeling?
   - What did you expect the food to do for you?
   - Was it a high-risk food?
   - Where were you eating? Were you engaged in another activity?

7) Determine what you can do next time to deal with the high risk situation:

√ Make a written plan so you have a visual guide for the next time.

√ Use new coping skills as alternatives to emotional eating.

√ Use Awareness Record and create a "recipe card" for each trigger. List alternative behavior (what you can do instead).

√ Avoid the trigger.

√ Seek support.

Determinants of Relapse

There has been significant research in the area of relapse prevention for addictions. (Brownell, Marlatt, Lichtenstein, and Wilson; Marlatt and Gordon, 1985; Turner, 1990; and Witkiewitz and Marlatt, 2004) have identified multiple factors that trigger and operate within high-risk situations and influence an individual's vulnerability to lapse and relapse. Their model incorporates the interaction between background factors (years of addiction, family history, co-morbid psychological conditions, and social support), physiological states, cognitive processes (self-efficacy, outcome expectancies, craving, the abstinence violation effect, and motivation), and coping skills.

- **Negative Emotional States**

    Stress and negative emotions weaken self-regulation (monitoring and altering one's behavior), thereby increasing risk of falling back into old patterns.

    What are you doing to manage your moods? _____

    _____

    _____

    _____

    _____

    _____

    _____

    _____

- **Poor Motivation**

  Do you remind yourself daily why you want your goal? _____

  _____

  _____

  _____

  _____

  What are you afraid of losing if you give up behaviors?

  Food/taste/pleasure _____

  _____

  _____

  Role of food _____

  _____

  _____

  _____

  Are you "just tired of it" — tired of the types of food you're eating, tired of planning,
  and tired of "dieting"? _____

  _____

  _____

  _____

If so, this is a good time to just take a break and plateau for a while. Even if you still want to lose more weight, taking a short break and focusing on weight maintenance will refresh you, and even give you a little boost in your metabolism. This is also a good opportunity to practice using *glow's* balance strategies – the Tier Approach, "planning and compensating," and Plan B to help you maintain your weight during this break. (You may need a couple of days, a week or two, or even a month.) When you feel ready, start with a reboot or reset.

- **Isolation/Poor Social Support**

  Be aware of social isolation. Isolation or loneliness can set you up for a relapse with addictive behavior. Are you involved in some type of support group/follow-up/after-care? _____

  _____

  _____

- **Interpersonal Conflicts**

  Do you feel equipped to resolve interpersonal issues? (Assertiveness, boundary setting, conflict resolution skills, etc.) _____

  _____

  _____

  _____

- **Physiological Factors**

  Are you managing conditions you were "self-medicating" with food? _____

  _____

  _____

  Is your goal weight realistic? (Set-point theory) _____

  _____

  _____

- **Misinterpreting Slips**

  Be mindful of how you talk to yourself after a slip. Be careful not to see the slip as a sign of personal weakness or failure but to attribute the slip to the external precipitating factors (which you can change!) Attacking yourself only undermines your self-worth and keeps you from assessing the situation.

Do you use cognitive restructuring to help you restore balance by using the Tier Approach or Planning and Compensating? _____

_____

_____

Abstinence Violation Effect (self-blame and loss of perceived control after violation of rule)

Replace negative thinking, i.e., "I overate, I blew it, and I will never be able to change... I may as well keep on eating" with cognitive restructuring (positive self-talk) i.e., a slip is a mistake; attribute to situation not self.

_____

_____

_____

It is not the slip that causes the relapse – it is how you respond to it.

- **Craving (Urge)**

Perceived availability plays a role in cravings. Are you managing your food cues? Are there some high-risk foods that should not be brought into the house at this time?

_____

_____

Urge surfing, a mindfulness technique attributed to Alan Marlatt, PhD (2004), can be useful for managing urges/cravings. An urge is like a wave. It rises in intensity, peaks, and then eventually subsides (usually within half an hour).

Exercise: Where in your body you are feeling the urge? Notice the sensation, but with non-judgment. Gently bring your attention to your breath. Use your breath to help you ride the wave like a surf board. Observe your breath as you ride out the wave. You don't have to act on an urge or do battle with it (which will just strengthen it). Just notice it, without judgment, and then gently bring your attention back to your breath.

- **Outcome Expectancy (Anticipation of the Effects of the Food)**

Positive expectancy increases food cravings. Are you able to use visualization or cognitive strategies to replace positive expectations (this will taste good, make me feel better, etc.) with negative expectations (this will spike my blood sugar, make me feel groggy, delay my goal, etc.)?

This concept is similar to identifying the pros/cons and deciding between instant gratification and your ultimate goal. Write down some statements that are specific for you.

_____

_____

_____

Remember to utilize your Awareness Record, Recipe Cards, and Bridge Flow Chart. What can I expect this food to do for me, and what else can I do instead? Is there a healthier alternative to eat?

_____

_____

_____

- **Pattern of "Testing the Boundaries of New Behavior"**

To maintain your weight-loss, you will not be able to go back to your original lifestyle; that is how the weight came on in the first place. This is where the concept of balance comes in. Have you learned how to eat and not overeat? Are you using the Tier Approach, and planning and compensating? Have you found balance?

_____

_____

_____

_____

_____

- **Out of Normal Routine: Major Stress/Loss, Vacation, Holiday, etc.**

  Be careful when it's "not business as usual" that you don't give yourself permission to eat with abandon. Be aware of your "diet mentality" and avoid falling into an "all or none" eating pattern. Again, this is a time to use balance strategies. Do you have a plan for high stress times?

  _____

  _____

  Plan for vacations/holidays _____

  _____

- **Self-Efficacy**

  Are you confident that you possess the coping skills and self-control strategies to manage stressful situations?

  Which of these skills do you feel confident in? Which of these skills do you need to develop or practice?

  √ Cognitive restructuring

  √ Emotional regulation

  √ Assertiveness/conflict resolution/boundary setting

  √ Expressing feelings/needs

  √ Journaling

  √ Relaxation/meditation/mindfulness

  √ Movement/physical activity

  √ Self-soothing

  √ Rest

  √ Leisure/recreation

  √ Spirituality

  √ Other_____

  _____

  _____

Additional Relapse Prevention Strategies

Awareness Record/Self-Monitoring

- Written plan
- Scheduled exercise
- Meal plan
- Shopping list
- Nutrition App
- Food/mood journal

Lifestyle Changes

Long-term relapse prevention involves a lifelong process of balancing work, relationships, spirituality, relaxation, exercise, rest, and leisure/recreation. There also is a need to balance self and others. Personal growth and insight into these areas will lead to greater self-efficacy and, ultimately, greater success in meeting your goals. It is helpful to occasionally assess if you are making time and scheduling time for these lifestyle changes that are meant to not only recharge you, but to provide a source of gratification that can replace the role that food is playing.

What plans do you have for balancing your work life? _____

_____

_____

_____

_____

_____

_____

_____

_____

What needs to happen to create balance in your personal relationships? *(Prioritize, boundaries, set limits, initiate, etc.)* _____

_____

_____

_____

_____

_____

_____

_____

_____

_____

What are your plans for exercise/movement? _____

_____

_____

_____

_____

What are your plans for relaxation/meditation? _____

_____

_____

_____

_____

What are your plans for rest/sleep? _____

_____

_____

_____

_____

What are your plans for balancing leisure time/recreation? _____

_____

_____

_____

_____

What areas need to be modified to create balance in nurturing self and nurturing relationships? _____

_____

_____

_____

_____

Preventative Measures (Increasing Stress Tolerance)

- Proper nutrition
- Regular exercise/movement
- Consistent relaxation/meditation practice
- Adequate sleep
- Social support
- Spiritual connection
- Self-nurturing behaviors

- Leisure/recreation
- Communicating feelings/needs

Plan for High-risk Situations

- **Visualization exercise:** Imagine yourself in a particularly difficult food situation, such as attending a party or eating at a restaurant. Visualize the scene in your mind and how you will handle the situation in a way that is consistent with your goals. For example, imagine that prior to the party, you have a non-caloric beverage and a serving of nuts. At the party you start with a non-alcoholic beverage and survey what food is being served. You probably started the day with the strategy of "planning" and have banked some calories. You take a small plate and start with your favorite fruits and vegetables, then a serving of protein, then a small serving of a special treat. If you decide to have an alcoholic beverage, you follow it with a glass of water. Repeat the visualization several times before the event.

- **Affirmations:** Carry written positive affirmations with you that you can look at throughout the day. These would be statements that motivate you and reaffirm your goals and your ability to reach them. For example:
  - "I am focusing on what my body needs today to be healthy."
  - "It's just a slip. What do I need to do now to compensate and get back on track?"
  - "A number on the scale does not determine my worth."
  - "I am fearfully and wonderfully made."
  - "It's not a diet; it's a lifestyle."
  - "It's all about balance."
  - "I am in charge of my life."
  - "I can do this!"
  -
  -
  -

Managing your Food/Weight Issues

Food/weight issues are best viewed as something you will "manage" the rest of your life. Many "recover" from emotional eating, but typically, if there has been a period of obesity, your body's physiology is primed for hanging on to those fat cells. Age and menopause also play a role in the physiological challenge of losing weight (fat). Environmental food cues will always be beckoning. Stress is an inevitable part of life. To top it all off, you cannot have complete abstinence from food. Thus, you may be free from emotional eating, but you may still have to "manage" your weight if weight-loss/maintenance is a goal.

Managing is a concept that we use with type 2 diabetes, allergies, anxiety, etc. Basically, if you follow the suggested guidelines, you can control your symptoms/condition. If you don't follow the guidelines, your symptoms will recur.

Managing does not mean dieting. It means learning how to eat and not overeat. It means learning how to incorporate your favorite foods – altering recipes and/or monitoring portion size or frequency of intake. Managing your food/weight means learning how to balance your food choices, as a healthy diet is one ingredient in effective weight management. You also need to incorporate exercise/movement and relaxation strategies, heal your emotional eating and body-image issues, challenge your diet-mentality, and change your response to food cues. Long-term weight management requires lifestyle changes.

This vital change in mindset will free you from the trap of chronic dieting and all of the patterns that are associated with it, including "all or none" thinking and behaviors, good food/bad food, restrict/binge...you get the idea.

A final note on body image: If you don't find peace with your body, you may continue to try to find the solution in dieting. Healing underlying body-image issues and learning to appreciate the body you have, can create the foundation for breaking free from compulsive dieting.

Strategies for Successful Weight-Loss Maintenance:

- *Keep a food journal (Awareness Record).*
- *Follow a written meal plan.*
- *Eat 3 meals a day at scheduled times.*
- *Eat breakfast (high protein).*
- *Include high-fiber foods.*
- *Drink at least 8 glasses of water a day.*
- *Reduce sugar and salt intake.*
- *Exercise regularly (not connected to whether or not you are "dieting").*
- *Monitor weight: have a "threshold" for weight re-gain to signal instituting self-correcting*

218

actions. Respond to small weight changes — depending on your body, water-weight, etc. Most people choose between 2-3 pound weight gain.

- *Have supportive relationships.*

- *Use positive self-talk.*

- *Attend a support group.*

- *Have reasonable expectations regarding weight-loss.*

- *Maintain a "diet," regardless of the stress in life.*

Chapter 7 Recap

√ See above list

√ Change your relationship with food

√ Change the role of food

√ Change "diet" mentality

√ Lifestyle changes

√ Use "balance" strategies – Tier approach, "planning and compensating," Plan B

√ Use Reset strategies to get back on track – Awareness record, journaling, meal planning, etc.

√ Continue to build coping skills

√ Practice relapse prevention skills

Journaling

Biopsychosocial Assessment

What are the changes you want to make at this time? _____

_____

_____

If weight-loss is one of your goals, what is your motivation (why do you want to lose weight)? _____

_____

_____

What, if anything, is holding you back? _____

_____

_____

Health Information

Medical conditions/illnesses: _____

_____

_____

Injuries/surgeries/hospitalizations: _____

_____

Pain or swelling: _____

Constipation, diarrhea, or gas: _____

For Women — Gynecological History

Any difficulty with menstrual cycle? _____ **PMS or menopausal issues?** _____

Birth Control History: _____

Food allergies or intolerance:_____

Diet restrictions (health or cultural): _____

Medications or supplements:_____

Family medical history: _____

_____

_____

How many hours per night do you sleep? _____ **Any disturbances in sleep?** _____

Caffeine Intake: _____ **Cigarette Use?** _____ *(Amount)* _____

Alcohol Use: _____*(Amount)* _____ *(Frequency)* _____

Drug Use? _____

History of alcohol or drug abuse/misuse/treatment? _____

Any other difficulties with impulse control (gambling, shopping, other)? _____

Mental health counseling/inpatient treatment? _____

Suicidal thoughts/attempts or self-harm behavior? _____

History of eating disorder (anorexia, bingeing, purging)?_____

Current mood (describe) _____

_____

_____

_____

Military history:_____

Legal history: _____

Family mental health history (including addictions):_____

_____

_____

_____

Food/Weight History

Height: _____   **Current weight:** _____

Highest weight: _____**When:** _____

Lowest weight at this height: _____**When:** _____

What is your ideal weight? _____

What is your level of body-image satisfaction?

Dislike Body   *Neutral*   *Like Body*

1   2   3   4   5   6   7   8   9   10

Please List Your Previous Attempts to Lose Weight:

Year	Method (Program, Medications, etc.)	Weight Lost	Comments (What worked well? What didn't work well?)

Do you eat when you are not hungry? Do you know what your triggers are? _____

_____

_____

Do you see yourself as an emotional eater? *(Do you use food to cope with negative feelings including stress, boredom, loneliness, procrastination, self-soothing?)* _____

Do you chronically restrict amount or types of food, but then when under stress, end up eating more than you normally would? _____

Do you have an "all or none" diet mentality *(good versus bad food, restrict or overeat)*? _____

Do you eat in front of the TV, while on your phone or computer, or while reading? _____

Do you feel like you need to eat a lot of food to feel full? _____

Do you have cravings? If so, what and when? _____

What foods did you eat as a child?

Breakfast _____

Lunch _____

Dinner _____

Snacks/Liquids _____

What is a typical day of eating, currently?

Breakfast _____

Lunch _____

Dinner _____

Snacks/Liquids _____

Describe your food/weight history: What do you attribute your food/weight issues to? _____

_____

_____

_____

_____

_____

What was the role of food/weight in your family of origin? _____

_____

_____

Were you raised in an environment where there was verbal, physical, or sexual abuse; neglect, alcoholism or drug abuse? _____

_____

_____

_____

Any other past traumas or losses? _____

Are you currently in an environment where there is any type of verbal, physical, or sexual abuse; or alcohol or drug abuse? _____

Will family/friends be supportive of your desire to make food and/or lifestyle changes? _____

List your support network: _____

_____

_____

What role does faith/spirituality play in your life? _____

_____

Describe your personality and level of self-esteem: _____

_____

_____

_____

How do you deal with stress or other negative emotions? _____

_____

Are you able to assert your feelings, needs, and boundaries? _____

How do you self-sooth and nurture yourself?_____

_____

What gives you pleasure in life?_____

_____

Are you currently experiencing any major life stressors? If so, how are you coping? _____

_____

_____

_____

Do you exercise? (Type and frequency): _____

_____

Do you do any type of relaxation strategies? _____

Is there anything else you would like to add that would help to personalize your plan? (Food preferences, budget, schedule, other family member) _____

_____

_____

How ready are you to make the changes that you are wanting, and what, if anything is holding you back? _____

_____

_____

get the glow

My Favorite Superfoods

I chose the following foods based on their nutrient content and health benefits, as well as for their direct or indirect impact on weight-loss. This is not intended to be a substitute for medication or a cure for any ailment. Please check with your medical provider to make sure none of the foods interact with medications or medical conditions.

Not surprising, most of the foods on the list are fruits and vegetables, including apples, avocados, beans (and other legumes), beets, berries (including blueberry, raspberry, and strawberry), cinnamon, cranberries, cruciferous vegetables (including cabbage, broccoli and cauliflower), dark chocolate, ginger, garlic, goji berries, green leafy vegetables (including kale and spinach), green tea, kombucha, mushrooms, nuts (including walnuts and almonds), oatmeal, olive oil, quinoa, salmon, seaweed, seeds (including chia and flax), and sweet potatoes.

Apples are high in fiber and polyphenols (antioxidant, anti-inflammatory, and fights bacteria in gut).

Avocados* are high in monosaturated fats and fiber (helps with satiety and cravings). They are high in magnesium (relaxing – helps with anxiety and sleep), lutein (eye health), potassium, betacarotene, and vitamins C, B6, and E (antioxidant and anti-inflammatory).

Beans* and other legumes are high in soluble fiber (stimulates CCK – satiety). They help lower cholesterol and decrease constipation. Beans contain antioxidants, folate, magnesium, iron, zinc, and choline (helps with focus and memory).

Beets are rich in betalains (a phytonutrient that is an antioxidant, anti-inflammatory, and a detoxifying agent; it is also know to help create red blood cells). Beets are also high in nitrates, a precursor to nitric oxide (increases blood flow, relaxes arteries, decreases blood pressure, artery plaque, and blood clotting).

Berries* are high in antioxidants – flavonoids, including quercetin (anti-inflammatory – helps with allergies, asthma, leaky gut, heart disease, and some cancers) and anthocyanins (anti-inflammatory which helps with memory, cognition, and motor function; and may decrease cell growth in some cancers).

Cinnamon* helps control insulin by decreasing blood sugar levels and helps with satiety by slowing digestion. It may also inhibit belly fat. Cinnamon contains antioxidants (polyphenal and flavonoid), is anti-inflammatory, and antimicrobial, thus, numerous health benefits including cardiac, neurological/cognitive, digestive, and immune system improvement, and may inhibit cell growth in some cancers.

Cranberries* are full of antioxidants, including anthocyanine. They are also anti-inflammatory and anti-bacterial, and may slow the cell growth of some cancers.

Cruciferous vegetables are anti-inflammatory and rich in antioxidants (glucosinolates) which have been shown to decrease the risk of cancer, especially lung, stomach, colon, liver, bladder, and breast. Contains sulfur compounds which supports collagen and keratin production for supple skin, strong hair, and nails.

Dark chocolate (70% cacao)* is anti-inflammatory and full of antioxidants. It is high in magnesium, increases dopamine, and decreases stress hormones. Cacao flavanols promote heart health by improving the elasticity of the blood vessels and lowering blood pressure, and improves cognitive function.

Ginger is anti-inflammatory and antimicrobial. It is known for its anti nausea effects. It may help with pain relief, cognitive decline, and fighting infection. It may curb hunger (the warm feeling in the stomach may help with feeling full). Ginger, along with cayenne, turmeric, green veggies, and oregano may help decrease amyloid plaque (residue from animals).

Garlic* has antioxidant, antibacterial, antifungal, antimicrobial, and antiviral properties. It is known to benefit the cardiovascular (lowering cholesterol, blood pressure, and regulating blood sugar) and immune systems. The sulfur compounds in garlic have been shown to lower the risk of certain cancers, especially upper gastrointestinal. Other vegetables in the allium family that contain the sulfur compounds include onions, leeks, chives, scallions, and shallots.

Goji berries* are high in fiber and chromium (which helps to control appetite by keeping blood sugar stable. It also helps to preserve muscle. These berries contains anti-inflammatory compounds (alpha linolenic and linoleic fatty acids) and antioxidants – betacarotene and lutein which promote healthy skin and immune function, and protects eye health; and lycopene which relaxes blood vessels and increases circulation. Goji berries also contain iron and protein.

Green leafy vegetables* including spinach, cabbage, lettuce, kale, bok choy, nappa cabbage, Swiss chard, collard and other greens are anti-inflammatory and contain antioxidants. Greens are very high in thylakoids, which promote the release of cholecystokinin (CCK), a hormone produced by the gastrointestinal tract that encourages a feeling of fullness. Greens help to alkalize the body, are high in fiber and chlorophyll (antioxidant, anti-cancer, liver detoxifier, and speeds up would healing). Dark greens also help repair DNA (methalation). Also high in vitamins A,C, E, K, folic acid, calcium, magnesium, iron, zinc, and potassium.

- Spinach – one cup is 12% of the RDA of calcium, and is high in vitamin K (beneficial to bone health, but also a natural blood thinner). Also high in lutein (protective against eye disease) and folate (beneficial to our blood, cells, and brain).

- Swiss chard is high in betalains (antioxidant, anti-inflammatory, and detoxifying agent), and is also high in vitamin K.
- Kale is high in carotenoids, flavonoids, iron, calcium, and vitamin K.

Green tea* is high in antioxidants; including polyphenols (free radical fighter), quercetin, and catechins (may inhibit belly fat). It also contains theanine which boosts alpha waves and promotes relaxation without sedation, increases GABA (anti-anxiety neurotransmitter), and increases dopamine (a neurotransmitter which promotes focus and concentration). Green tea provides an alert, mental calm. Health benefits may also include decreasing the risk of diabetes, Alzheimers, some cancers (angiogenesis inhibitor), cardiovascular disease, and bacterial infections.

Kombucha is a lightly effervescent fermented tea that is full of probiotics.

Mushrooms are full of antioxidants, selenium, B vitamins, and vitamin D. They are known for boosting the immune system. There are many varieties that are used for medicinal purposes, including fighting cancer (they are categorized as an angiogenesis inhibitor, which prevents abnormal cells from obtaining blood to grow). The shiitake mushroom is a commonly known gourmet mushroom that is also considered medicinal.

Nuts* are a good source of protein, healthy fat, and fiber. Monosaturated fats trigger CCK. Part of a heart healthy diet, may lower cholesterol.

- Walnuts are high in omega 3 fatty acids, which help to regulate ghrelin and leptin (hunger and satiety hormones). Omega 3 fatty acids are anti-inflammatory and strengthen the immune system. They also effect dopamine and serotonin transmission and have a role in brain development and functioning; deficiencies have been linked to mental health problems such as depression, anorexia nervosa, and ADHD. Walnuts are also high in vitamin E.
- Almonds are the most nutritionally dense nut. A serving provides 50% of the RDA of vitamin E, 8% RDA of calcium, and also contain potassium, magnesium, and iron.
- Cashews provide 26% RDA of magnesium (relaxes muscles and mood, and increases insulin sensitivity so may slash diabetes risk by almost half), and also zinc and selenium, which enhance the immune system.
- Brazil nuts contain 100% RDA of selenium in just one nut. Selenium may play a role in breast cancer prevention.
- Hazel nuts are high in the antioxidant proanthocyonidins (strengthens blood vessels and may prevents UTI's); iron, and folate (may help with depression and heart disease).
- Pistachios contain sterols which may help lower cholesterol. These nuts are also high in potassium.

- Pecans provide magnesium (antioxidant and anti-inflammatory), manganese (anti-inflammatory), vitamins A, E, zinc, and folate (which are all great for your skin), L-arganine (promotes hair growth and flexible arterial walls), oleic acid (a monosaturated fat that may decrease the risk of breast cancer), ellaic acid (may slow the growth of some cancers and may help liver neutralize carcinogenic chemicals, is antibacterial and antiviral).

Oatmeal* (steel-cut oats) is high in fiber and antioxidant. This whole-grain has been shown to lower cholesterol levels, help with constipation, and stabilize blood sugar. Also high in biotin, which promotes radiant skin, shiny hair, and strong nails.

Olive oil (extra virgin)* is high in omega 3 fatty acids and oleic acid (both anti-inflammatory). A serving provides 72% RDA of vitamin E and 75% RDA of vitamin K.

Quinoa is high in protein (8 grams per one-cup serving). Quinoa is one of the only grains or seeds that provide all nine essential amino acids our bodies can't produce themselves.

Salmon* is high in omega 3 fatty acids (anti-inflammatory) which may help reduce the risk of cardiovascular disease. It is also high in vitamin D3, which is thought to help with immune function, and decrease risk for depression, diabetes, osteoporosis, obesity, and some cancers. Salmon may also protect skin from the sun and the damaging effects of UV rays.

Sea vegetables/algae*

- Seaweed (kelp, nori, etc.), is high in nutrients but low in calories. The benefits of seaweed include strengthening of mucus that protects the wall of the gut, prevention of high blood pressure, detoxification properties that may aid the body in fighting cancer, and regulation of hormones. It is high in vitamins C, A, B6, and fiber. Used for heavy metal detox. Some seaweeds are high in iodine (may need to monitor this if you have a thyroid condition).
- Spirulina is freshwater, blue - green algae that is a complete protein (65%), vitamins A, K, B12, iron, manganese, chromium, and betacarotene. It is being used for heavy metal detox, as antimicrobial to treat candida, and may play a role in cancer prevention, lowering blood pressure and cholesterol, and decreasing arterial plaque.

Seeds*, including chia, flax, hemp, sunflower, pumpkin, and sesame, are high in protein, fiber, and healthy fat. Seeds provide satiety and help balance blood sugar.

- Chia seeds are high in omega 3 fatty acids (anti-inflammatory). Chia seeds are a complete protein, and are high in magnesium, iron, calcium, and potassium. These seeds absorb 10 times their weight in liquid to help you feel full and stay full longer.
- Flax seed (ground) is high in omega 3 fatty acids and lignans (phytoestrogens, which may decrease breast and other hormone sensitive cancer risk). It may even help to reduce belly fat.

- Hemp is a complete protein, high in omega 3's, iron, vitamin E, and magnesium.

- Sesame seeds are high in polyphenals (lignans), calcium, magnesium, iron, zinc, and selenium.

- Pumpkin seeds are high in antioxidants, betacarotene, a precursor to vitamin A, which is known for its immune boosting powers and role in eye health.

Turmeric is an anti-inflammatory and antioxidant that may help decrease the risk of Alzheimers, depression, and the growth of some cancers.

* Most of these superfoods contain antioxidants, omega 3's, or other phytonutrients that have been shown to help promote radiant skin and shiny hair – to "get the *glow*."

Notes

Healthy Snacks (Ideas for Craving Substitutions)

Most of these snacks are protein, healthy fat, or fiber based. When you are craving something specific in flavor, texture, or temperature that is not a healthy choice and you are wanting to refrain from eating it (at this moment in time) try to substitute with a food that is similar to what you are craving, e.g., salty, sweet, savory, tart, crunchy, creamy, etc.

Savory or Salty Craving:

- Layered Greek dip: Hummus, Greek yogurt, minced garlic, cucumber, tomato, Kalamata olives, and feta cheese. Use for dipping vegetables (carrots, cauliflower, cucumbers, peppers, zucchini, jicama, etc.) or whole grain/lentil/black bean crackers – creamy and crunchy

- Olive tapenade and/or hummus with crudités or healthy crackers – creamy and crunchy

- Olives and baby bell or string cheese – creamy

- Deviled egg (use plain Greek yogurt and mustard) – creamy

- Edamame with sea salt – creamy

- Roasted edamame – crunchy

- Popcorn, pop in coconut oil – crunchy

- Roasted sweet potato chips – crunchy

- Roasted kale chips – crunchy

- Roasted seaweed snacks – crunchy

- Roasted chickpeas – crunchy

- Guacamole and salsa with wholegrain tortilla chips – crunchy

- Turkey jerky – chewy

Sweet and Creamy Craving:

- Chocolate, peanut butter and banana shake: frozen banana, 1 tbsp. peanut butter, 1 tbsp. cocoa powder, 1/2 c. vanilla almond milk – blend.

- Frozen banana-chocolate drops: cut banana into one inch slices; dip in melted dark chocolate (optional – top with chopped nuts) or try adding a smear of peanut butter before dipping in the chocolate. Place on waxed paper, freeze, then place in freezer bag.

- Chia pudding: basic recipe – 1 c. unsweetened almond, cashew, or coconut milk, 1/4 c. chia seeds, 1/8 tsp. vanilla (optional). Add all ingredients to a glass container, stir, cover, and refrigerate for at least 2-4 hours or overnight. Additional add-ins to try: cinnamon, bananas, figs, dates, raisins, berries, mango, citrus zest, dark chocolate shavings, shredded coconut, etc.

- Strawberries, bananas, pears dipped in melted dark chocolate
- Dark chocolate and nut drops (melt 1 oz. dark chocolate, add 1/2 oz. nuts)
- Frozen grapes (popsicle substitute) or frozen raisins/figs/prunes (kind of caramel-like)
- Baked apple or sweet potato with cinnamon and chopped walnuts or pecans (optional – top with yogurt)
- Flavored Greek yogurt, with fruit and/or nuts

Chewy:

- Raisins, goji berries, dried fruit (in moderation as it has a high sugar content)
- Jerky

Crunchy:

- Raw vegetables with dips made from hummus, yogurt, salsa, or tahini.
- Apple slices, nut butter optional
- See above under Savory/Salty

Sweet and Salty:

- Trail mix with nuts, raisins, and dark chocolate chips
- Dark chocolate nut drops (see above)
- Watermelon with feta, sprinkled with balsamic vinegar and basil leaves

Awareness Record
Stop • Breathe • Reflect • Listen to Your Inner Voice

Why do I want to make lifestyle changes?

Today's Goal?

Differentiate Between Physical Hunger and Psychological Triggers
(Physiological, Emotional, Diet-mentality, or Environmental cues)

- Am I physically hungry? Am I thirsty?

- Is there an external cue?

Change the Role of Food *(Health Focus)*

- How will this food nourish my body?

- How does this food make my body feel physically/mentally?

Food/Mood Journal

Explore your Emotional Eating

What are you feeling? What do you need?

- What do you expect the food to do for you?

- How can you deal with it in a healthy way? (Alternative coping strategies)

Are you trying to avoid anything?

- If so, what are your fears?

- If you decide to not deal with it right now, what are healthy "avoidance strategies"?

What is your self-talk?

- Do you need to challenge it with cognitive restructuring?

Daily Awareness Record

Time *(Meal/Snack)*	Nutrition *(Amount)*	Level of Hunger/Satiety *(Internal Cues)* *(Rate 1–10)*	Trigger(s) *(External Cues)* *(Location, Activity, Mood, Self-Talk)*	Comments

Water Intake
(O = 1 cup) O O O O
O O O O

Movement: **Relaxation:**   **Self-Care:**

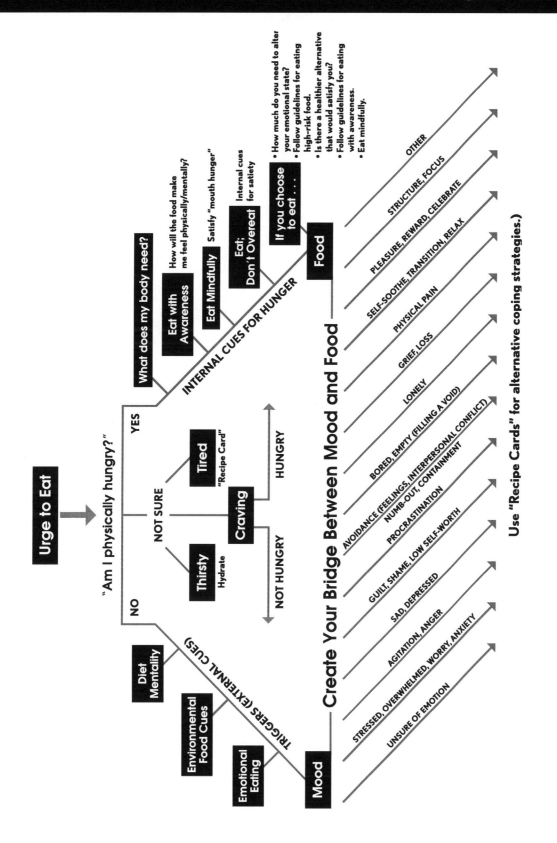

Create Your Bridge Between Mood and Food

239

Unsure of Emotion(s)

- Relaxation strategy to decrease SNS
- Journaling or column technique to externalize emotions and increase insight
- Cognitive restructuring
- Social support to provide reflective listening
- Emotional regulation strategies
-
-
-
-
-
-
-

--------✂------- -

Stressed/Overwhelmed/Worry, Anxiety

- Relaxation strategies to decrease SNS, increase PNS
  - Diaphragmatic breathing
  - Meditation, including MBSR
- Physical release – movement/exercise
- Column technique to sort out issues/feelings
- Journaling to externalize feelings and gain awareness
- Social support
- Cognitive restructuring
- Time-management strategies
- Restorative practices - leisure/recreation
- Warm bath
- Nap   •
- Delegate, say "no"   •

Agitated, Angry

- Time-out – to de-escalate physically and emotionally
- Decrease SNS arousal
  - Relaxation strategies (including slow, deep breaths)
  - Movement/exercise
- Emotional regulation strategies (including DBT)
- Journal feelings
- Use cognitive restructuring
- Social and/or spiritual support
-
-
-
-

✂ —

Sad, Depressed

- Journal and cognitive restructuring
- Social and/or spiritual support
- Self-soothing/self-care strategies
- Listen to uplifting music
- Gratitude journal
- Pleasurable activity – use creativity, stimulate sense of humor
- Volunteer – help someone in need
- Pet therapy
-
-
-
-

Guilt/Shame, Low Self-Worth

- Cognitive restructuring
- Positive affirmations
- Self-compassion strategies
- Spirituality/self-forgiveness
- Social support
-
-
-
-
-
-
-

✂ —

Procrastination (Avoidance)

- Third option – healthy avoidance alternatives
- Include indoor, outdoor, solitary, and social options
- Pick options that last 15-30 minutes, to give you a short break but also remind you that you probably need to address what you are avoiding.
- Build skills to decrease procrastination (write out plan; break it down into small parts, etc.) If this is a pattern, may need to rule out perfectionism or ADD/ADHD
-
-
-
-
-
-

Avoidance of Feelings or Issues/Numb-Out

- Healthy avoidance alternatives
  - Read a magazine or book
  - Go for a walk
  - Meditate
  - Watch TV or a movie
  - Play a game on computer/phone
  - Call a friend
  - Tap into spirituality
  - Rest, nap
  -
  -
  -
- Journal and utilize cognitive restructuring to explore issue and fear of dealing with it

 —

Containment/Grounding

- Utilize therapeutic strategies for containment and grounding
- Utilize safe place imagery
- Use "wrapping" technique (roll self up in a blanket)
- Diaphragmatic breathing
- Utilize touch – texture
- Rub lotion on arms
- Color, draw, paint
- Rock back and forth in a rocking chair
-
-
-
-

Bored

- Assess if there is another feeling that is actually present – empty, lonely, avoidance of feelings.
- Pleasurable activity or hobby
- Connect – social, spiritual
- Go to a park/spend time in nature
- Do craft, art, dance, listen to music
- Give yourself a manicure or pedicure
- Color – adult coloring book
- Read
- Ride bike, go for a walk
-
-

✂ —

Lonely, Empty

- Reach out to support system – call, text, email
  Who can you call
- Increase connections – social, spiritual
- Plan weekly social activities
- Volunteer
- Join an organization, class, group
- If fear is stopping you from meeting people, you may need to rule-out social anxiety. If you feel empty, what is missing in your life?
-
-
-
-

Grief/Loss

- Allow yourself to feel the feelings
- Journal feelings and use cognitive restructuring if needed (for irrational guilt)
- Wrap yourself in a blanket
- Reach out to support system (grief is not meant to do alone)
- Spiritual practices – prayer, scripture, etc.
- Join a support group
- Spend time in nature or have an "awe" experience
- Volunteer
-
-
-
-

Chronic Pain

- Utilize pain management strategies (Jon Kabot-Zinn's *Full Catastrophe Living* is a great resource)
- Utilize self-soothing activities (warm bath, aromatherapy, music)
- Use heating pad or ice packs
- Utilize self-massage
- Relaxation strategies – breathing, yoga, gentle stretching
- Engage senses for distraction
- Schedule massage, acupuncture, etc. per provider
- Rest, nap
-
-
-

Self-Soothing, Transition (After Work or After Kids in Bed), Relaxation

- Sensual experiences (target your 5 senses)
  - Bubble bath with lavender bath salts, candles, soft music, etc.
  - Aromatherapy
  - Massage, manicure/pedicure
- Listen to music, watch TV, read (do not pair with eating, but okay to have a soothing drink – hot tea, flavored water, or a kombucha)
- Relaxation strategies – meditation, yoga
- Restorative practices, leisure activities
- Rest, nap
-
-
-
-

- -

Pleasure, Celebration, Reward ("I deserve...")

- What else is pleasurable and/or rewarding to you?
-
-
-
- Some of the items from Self-soothing may apply (sensual experiences)
-
-
-
- Positive affirmations
- Social connection
-
-

Structure, Focus

- Utilize column technique
- Utilize day planner, schedule, lists
- Mindful meditation and other breathing techniques
- Grounding strategies
-
-
-
-
-
-
-
-

✂ —

Interpersonal Issues

- Journal feelings
- Assertive communication
- Boundaries and limit setting
- Conflict resolution skills
- Utilize healthy avoidance strategies if choosing to not deal with the issue at the moment
-
-
-
-
-
-

Fatigue/Low Energy

- Assess if you really need to stay awake or is it time to take a break, rest or go to bed.
- If you need to stay awake for a bit, but don't want the added stimulation of caffeine, then try
  - 10 minutes of stair climbing or other aerobic activity
  - A brisk walk outside (weather and time of day permitting)
  - A glass of cold water (dehydration often causes low energy)
  - Opening a window for fresh, cool air
- Listen to your body; it may be time to take a break.
  - Restorative practices
  - Yoga, meditation, relaxation strategies
  - Catnap (20 minutes)
- Is it bedtime? Go to bed! (It's okay.)
-
-

Other

-
-
-
-
-
-
-
-
-
-
-

Other

-
-
-
-
-
-
-
-
-
-
-
-

- -

Other

-
-
-
-
-
-
-
-
-
-
-
-

Emotional Health Screen

This screen is not intended to be used for diagnosis or treatment. This is a preliminary tool, designed to increase awareness of co-occurring symptoms that may be interfering with emotional eating and/or weight loss efforts. If the symptoms are persistent, and interfere with daily functioning, they may be part of a mental- health or medical condition. Please consult with your provider for an accurate diagnosis.

Do you

- Binge-eat
  - √ Eating in a short period of time, an amount that is larger than most people would eat.
  - √ Loss of control over how much you are eating.
  - √ Eat much more rapidly than normal
  - √ Eat until uncomfortably full.
  - √ Feel upset with yourself after overeating.

- Engage in compensatory behaviors to prevent weight gain (including self-induced vomiting, laxative abuse, fasting, or excessive exercise)?

Are you

- A worrier
  - √ Do you find it difficult to control the worry?
  - √ Do you have trouble falling or staying asleep?
  - √ Do you have trouble concentrating?
  - √ Do you have trouble with irritability?

- Do you experience physical symptoms of anxiety?
  - √ Do you experience muscle tension, headaches, stomach aches, or diarrhea?
  - √ Do you bite your nails, pick your cuticles, or bite the inside of your cheeks?
  - √ Are you easily fatigued?
  - √ Do you have racing or pounding of your heart?
  - √ Do you feel restless or shaky?
  - √ Have you ever used alcohol or drugs to "take the edge off"?

Have you

- Felt depressed, sad, or "flat," more days than not, for at least 2 years?

√ Do you experience insomnia or want to sleep a lot?

√ Do you experience low energy?

√ Do you have low self-esteem?

√ Do you feel hopeless?

Have you experienced these symptoms consistently for 2 weeks or more?

- Sad/depressed mood or "flat"
- Little interest or pleasure in doing things
- Thought of death or suicide
- Self-critical
- Poor concentration, difficulty making decision
- Low energy, decreased motivation
- Irritability, restless
- Sleep disturbances (insomnia or hypersomnia)

Has there ever been a period of time when you were not your usual self and

- Your mood was elevated, irritable, or "too cheerful"?

    √ You had more energy than normal or felt hyper?

    √ Your mind was racing and you felt a need to talk a lot?

    √ You were more social or outgoing?

    √ You needed much less sleep, but still felt rested?

    √ You were more impulsive or engaged in risky behavior (financial, sexual, or other)?

    √ You felt grandiose or self-esteem was inflated?

    √ You experienced "mood swings"?

    √ Felt like you needed to use alcohol or drugs to calm yourself down?

Were you diagnosed with ADD or ADHD as a child or do you have a child who is diagnosed with ADD/ADHD?

Are you

- Easily distracted, have difficulty focusing or paying attention?

    √ Do you have trouble following through on projects?

    √ Are you forgetful or do you have trouble losing things?

√ Do you avoid tasks that require sustained mental effort?

√ Are you disorganized – with things and time?

√ Do you procrastinate?

- Impulsive?

  √ Do you have difficulty with interrupting others or waiting your turn?

  √ Do you speak without thinking?

  √ Do you make decisions before thinking through the consequences?

  √ Do you engage in risky or compulsive behaviors (alcohol, drugs, gambling sexual activity, over-spending, or shoplifting)?

- Do you feel like you always need to keep moving or be doing something?

  √ Do you have difficulty remaining quiet, talking too loudly or excessively?

  √ Do you feel physically restless?

  √ Do you have difficulty with leisure activity or just relaxing?

Have you ever had any experience that was so frightening, that you

- Have nightmares or experienced intrusive memories about it?

- Have "flashbacks" (feel that the event is happening in the here and now)?

- Go out of your way to avoid situations that reminded you of it?

- Have difficulty remembering parts of the experience?

- Use alcohol, drugs, or food to "numb-out"?

Are you

√ Constantly on guard or easily startled?

√ Self-destructive or have negative beliefs about yourself?

Do you

√ Feel numb or detached from others, activities, or your surroundings?

√ Have difficulty with irritability or anger outbursts, easily stressed, or over-reactive?

√ Have sleep disturbances?

Do you experience any of these symptoms as a consistent part of your life?

- Severe mood swings

- Rage or temper outbursts

- Extreme changes in how you see yourself (from self-confident to worthless)
- Feelings of emptiness
- Major shifts in your opinions about others (love/hate)
- Intense, volatile relationships
- Fears of abandonment and going to extremes to keep someone from leaving you
- Risky, impulsive, or self-destructive behavior (alcohol, drugs, sex, over-spending, etc.)
- Self-harm or suicidal behavior
- Sense of detachment from reality

Please remember that this is not a diagnostic instrument. If you have questions or concerns about any of the symptom clusters that you may see yourself in, please contact your medical provider.

Ideas for Menu Planning

Breakfast (high protein)

Frittata: (eggs, minced garlic, sliced mushroom or zucchini, shredded cheese, herbs, kale – on top; serve with sliced avocado). Make on Sunday for brunch – leftovers for next day's breakfast, lunch, or dinner.

Omelet or Egg "muffins": make mini-omelet's in muffin tins (add veggies, meat, etc.).

Hard boiled eggs – reheat or eat cold.

Protein Smoothie: protein powder, 1/2 c. spinach (I keep a bag in the freezer), 1/2 c. frozen berries, 1/2 frozen banana, 1-2 tbsp. chia/flax blend, 1/2-3/4 c. vanilla almond milk.

Steel-cut oatmeal with walnuts and or seeds (chia, flax, sunflower, or pumpkin): Overnight oatmeal (Crockpot or refrigerator version)

Banana with peanut or nut butter.

Whole wheat toast with peanut butter, topped with blueberries/strawberries, add a drizzle of honey (optional) or home-made chia "jam."

Greek yogurt with chia/flax seed, chopped nuts, and berries.

Whole grain toast with sliced avocado, sprinkled with sesame seeds.

Lunch (high protein)

Build a Salad:

- Alternate different types of greens (romaine, bibb, kale, spinach, arugula, radicchio) or use broccoli slaw, coleslaw, bok choy, or napa cabbage as a base.
- Pile on more vegetables (peppers, mushrooms, onions, shredded carrots, cauliflower, broccoli, shredded brussel sprouts, jicama, radishes, cucumber, roasted or canned beets, peapods, etc.).
- Add protein (chicken or turkey breast, precooked shrimp, salmon or tuna, hard-boiled eggs, legumes (beans) – garbanzo, black, peas, lentils, edamame, etc.).
- Add a healthy fat (avocado, olives, chopped nuts –pecans, walnuts, almonds, cashews or seeds –sunflower, pumpkin, etc.).
- Make a healthy dressing (with olive or walnut oil as a base, add balsamic or other vinegar

or lemon or lime juice, and choice of spice or herb – garlic, Dijon mustard, ginger, etc.). You can also use avocado, yogurt, soy-sauce, tahini , salsa, etc. as a base for a blended dressing.

- Optional:
  - Add fruit (tomatoes, berries, apples, pears, orange segments, grapes, etc.).
  - Add cheese (parmesan, feta, goat, ricotta or cottage, etc.).

- Chicken salads (serve on a bed of greens):
  - Curried chicken almond: Cooked chicken, sliced almonds and celery, and sliced hard-boiled egg. Toss with Greek yogurt mixed with curry.
  - Cashew Chicken: Cooked chicken breast, mandarin orange slices, cashew halves, scallions, and peapods. Toss with a sesame-ginger dressing.
  - Pecan Chicken: 2 c. cooked chicken, ½ c. pecan pieces, 1 c. grape halves, and ½ c. chopped celery. Toss with ½ c. Greek yogurt and 1 tbsp honey.

- Tuna/Salmon salads (serve on a bed of greens):
  - Apple/walnut tuna salad: mix can/pack of tuna with 1/4 c. Greek yogurt, add ¼ c. finely chopped apple, ¼ c. chopped walnuts; top with sliced black olives, sunflower seeds, and shredded mozzarella (optional). Drizzle with raspberry vinaigrette.
  - Salmon/or Tuna Nicoise: I use a pack of tuna or salmon for this; add sliced hard- boiled egg, sliced Bermuda onion, blanched green beans, Nicoise or Kalamata olives, capers, and cherry tomatoes. Drizzle with olive oil/lemon juice vinaigrette (2 tbsp walnut or olive oil, 1 tbsp juice, minced garlic clove, and ¼ tsp anchovy paste (optional).
  - Tuna, salmon, or precooked salad shrimp and avocado boat: ½ avocado, top with fish or shrimp. Top with salsa.

- Egg Salad: Add capers and black olives; mix with Greek yogurt, mustard, celery salt.

- Taco salad: Use seasoned ground turkey/beef or make it vegetarian. Add avocado, black olives, black beans, lettuce, tomatoes or salsa, shredded cheese (optional), and top with Greek yogurt mixed with salsa, lime juice, and cumin. Sprinkle with fresh cilantro.

For variety, some of the above salads would pair well on whole grain bread or mixed with a whole grain (brown rice, quinoa, etc.).

Plan B Time-Savers

- Crock pot or pressure cooker recipes

- Stir-fry's – buy precut or cut veggies night before

- Use Simple recipes with for most of your meals during the week. If the protein entrée requires extra ingredients, go for a Simple vegetable side-dish. Save experimenting with new recipes or recipes with a list of ingredients for the weekend.

- Double up a recipe to have leftovers for lunch the next day or to use in another dish.

  Example: Fresh salmon, brown rice and broccoli the night before can become salmon patties or a rice bowl the next day. Flake the salmon, add to rice and chopped broccoli (add additional stir fried vegetable if you'd like), add soy sauce/tamari, wasabi paste and reheat, top with roasted seaweed (optional).

  Example: I often use canned salmon for a rice bowl (above) for dinner and the next day for lunch use the leftover rice and salmon for a "cold bowl." Flake the salmon, add rice, chopped avocado, chopped cucumber, thinly sliced radish or green onion, soy or tamari sauce, wasabi paste, and roasted seaweed (yum! – one of my favorites!)

Example of a Simple Meal:

- Roasted chicken breast with garlic and tarragon:

  Smooth 1 tsp of coconut oil in bottom of baking dish, place chicken in dish, sprinkle with garlic powder and dried tarragon, salt optional. Bake chicken breasts at 450 for 20 minutes.

- Steamed broccoli (sprinkle with shredded parmesan)

- Quinoa (optional) – you can make ahead or use the microwave quick pack.

Example of Simple Meal (vegetarian):

- Spaghetti Squash with Marinara or Pesto
- Tossed Green Salad
- Watermelon Salad with Feta and Basil

Example of a Simple Meal:

- Grilled salmon with lemon slices and dill
- Stir-fried vegetables (frozen or pre-cut) with soy sauce, minced garlic, and sesame oil
- Brown rice (optional) – make ahead or use microwave quick pack

Example of a Simple Meal:

- Crockpot Turkey breast with sage and thyme
- Sweet Potatoes (add to Crockpot or microwave)
- Green beans (canned, frozen, or steamed)

Example of a Simple Meal:

- Grilled steak
- Grilled veggie kabobs – onion, pepper, mushrooms, etc. brush with olive oil and garlic powder
- Grilled red potatoes with olive oil and minced garlic and rosemary (cube potatoes and wrap in tinfoil) – (optional)

Example of a Simple Meal:

- Fish tacos (poach halibut, tilapia, cod in ½ c. coconut milk or pan fry in 1 tbsp coconut oil)
- Serve with shredded cabbage, sliced radishes, sliced avocado, black beans
- Corn tortillas and shredded cheese (optional)
- Top with Salsa, Greek yogurt mixed with 1 tsp lime juice and ½ tsp cumin, and fresh cilantro

Example of a Simple Meal:

- Grilled or fried hamburger
- Roasted potatoes (cut up like fries, toss with olive oil, garlic, sea salt, and rosemary)
- Tossed green salad loaded with veggies
- Yep, that's right; you can eat this if you want to. You may choose to have grass-fed beef, and/or you can choose to skip the bun if you are going to have the potatoes. Remember, the key is Balance – Planning and Compensating and using the Tier Approach. It is your plan.

What are a couple of simple meals you could add to this list to have for a quick reference?

- _____

  _____

- _____

  _____

References

Agras, W.S. (1987). *Eating disorders: management of obesity, bulimia, and anorexia nervosa.* New York, NY: Pergamon.

Amen, G. (2011). *The Amen solution: The brain healthy way to get thinner, smarter, and happier.* New York, NY: Three Rivers Press.

American Psychiatric Association. (2013). *Diagnostic and Statistical Manual of Mental Disorders, (5th Ed.).* Washington, DC: American Psychiatric Publishing.

Bailey, M.T., Dowd, S.E., Galley, J.D., Hufnagle, A.R., Allen, R.G., & Lyte, M. (2011). Exposure to a social stressor alters the structure of intestinal microbiota: Implications for stressor-induced immunomodulation. Brain, Behavior, and Immunity.

Beck, A.T. (1976). *Cognitive therapy and emotional disorders.* New York, NY: International University Press.

Benson, H. (1998). *Mind-body medicine: Clinical perspective and update.* Presented by Harvard Medical School; Marco Island, Florida.

Blass, E. (2008). *Obesity: Causes, mechanisms, prevention, and treatment.* Sinauer Associates: Sunderland, MA.

Blum, K., Braverman, E.R., Holder, J.M., Lubar, J.O., Monastra, V.J., Miller, D., Chen, T.J.H., and Comings, D.E. (2000). The reward deficiency syndrome: A biogenic model for the diagnosis and treatment of impulsive, addictive, and compulsive behaviors. *Journal of Psychoactive Drugs*, 32, 1-112.

Boskind-Lodahl, M. (1981). Cinderella's stepsisters: A feminist perspective on anorexia and bulimia. In Howell, I. & Bayes, H. (EDs.) *Women and Mental Health.* New York, NY: Basic Books, Inc.

Bowers, D. (2005). *Traumatic stress, PTSD, and grief.* Workshop presented by PESI, Sioux Falls, SD.

Brewerton, T. (2007). Eating disorders, trauma, and comorbidity: Focus on PTSD. *Eating disorders,* 15, 285-304.

Brownell, K.D., Marlatt, F.A., Lichtenstein, E., & Wilson, G.T. (1986). *Understanding and preventing relapse.* American Psychologist, 41 (7), 765-782.

Bruch, H. (1973). Eating disorders: *Obesity, anorexia nervosa, and the person within.* New York, NY: Basic Books.

Bruch, H. (1978). *The golden cage: The enigma of anorexia nervosa.* Cambridge: Harvard University Press.

Buettner, D. (2008). *The blue zone: Lessons for living longer, from the people who've lived the longest.* National Geographic Society: Washington, DC.

Callahan, L. (2002). *The fitness factor: Every woman's key to a lifetime of health and well-being.* Guilford, CT: Lyons Press.

Cash, T. F. (1990). *Body-image enhancement: A program for overcoming negative body image.* New York, NY: Guilford.

Cash, T.F. (2008). *The body-image workbook: An eight step program for learning to like your looks.* Oakland, Ca: New Harbinger Publications.

Chernin, K. (1983). *Womansize: The tyranny of slenderness.* London: Women's Press.

Chernin, K. (1986). *The hungry self: Women, eating, and identity.* New York, NY: Harper and Row.

Cochrane, C.E., Brewerton, T.D., Wilson, D.B., Hodges, E.L. (1993). Adaptive functions of eating disorder symptoms. *International Journal of Eating Disorders,* 14 (2), 219-222.

Coker Ross, C. (2016). *The emotional eating workbook: A proven-effective, step-by-step guide to end your battle with food and satisfy your soul.* Oakland, CA: New Harbinger Publications.

Colbert, D. (2016). *Let food be your medicine: Dietary changes proven to prevent or reverse disease.* Franklin, TN: Worthy Books.

Colino, S. (2014). The sound of healing. *Alternative medicine: Your guide to stress relief, healing, nutrition, and more.* New York, NY: Time Books.

Cottone, P., Sabino, V., Steardo, L., & Zorrilla, E.P. (2008). Intermittent access to preferred food reduces the reinforcing efficacy of chow in rats. Am J Physiol Regul Integr Comp Physiol. Oct; 295(4):R1066-76.

Craighead, L, (2006). *The appetite awareness workbook: How to listen to your body and overcome bingeing, overeating, and obsession with food.* Oakland, CA: New Harbinger Publications.

Crisp, A. (1981). Anorexia nervosa at a normal body weight - the abnormal normal weight control syndrome. I*nternational Journal of Psychiatry in Medicine,* 11, 203-233.

Crisp, A. H. & Kalucy, R.S. (1974). Aspects of the perceptual disorder in anorexia nervosa. *British Journal of Medical Psychology,* 47, 349-361.

Dossey, L. (1993). *Healing words: The power of prayer and the practice of medicine.* New York, NY: HarperCollins

Ehrenreich, B. & English, D. (1978). *For her own good: 150 years of the expert's advice to women.* New York, NY: Anchor Press/Doubleday.

Erikson, E. (1968). *Identity: Youth and crisis.* New York, NY: Norton.

Epstein, P. (2015). *Mind-body medicine.* Lecture [online], Institute for Integrative Nutrition.

Faelten, E. (Ed.), (1996). *Food and you: Everything a woman needs to know about loving food – for better health, for a beautiful body, and for emotional satisfaction.* Emmaus, Pennsylvania: Rodale Press Inc.

Fairburn, C.G. (1985). Cognitive-behavioral treatment for bulimia. In D.M. Garner & P.E. Garfinkel (EDs.) *Handbook of psychotherapy for anorexia nervosa and bulimia,* (pp.160-192). New York, NY: Guilford Press.

Foley-Henry, R. (2014). How to keep your mind sharp. *Alternative medicine: Your guide to stress relief, healing, nutrition, and more.* New York, NY: Time Books.

Freedman, R. (1986). *Beauty bound.* Lexington, MA: D.C. Health.

Gay, P. (1997). *Ego state therapy with eating disorders.* Workshop, Two Rivers Psychiatric Hospital, Kansas City, MS.

Gregory-bills, T. (1990). *Eating disorders and their correlates in earlier episodes of incest.* Doctoral dissertation. University of Houston.

Harvard Health Publications, (2015). Glycemic index and glycemic load for 100 + foods. http://www.health.harvard.edu/diseases-and-conditions/the-lowdown-on-glycemic-index-and-glycemic-load.

Hayes, S.C., Stroshal, K., & Wilson, K.G. (1999). *Acceptance and Commitment therapy: An experiential approach to behavior change.* New York, NY: Guilford Press.

Herbert, B.M., Blechert, J., Hautzinger, M., Matthias. E., Herbert, C. (2013). Intuitive eating is associated with interoseptive sensitivity: Effects on body mass index. *Appetite,* 11 (70), 22-30.

Herman, C.P. & Polivy, J. (1975). Anxiety, restraint, and eating behavior. *Journal of Abnormal Psychology*, 84 (6), 666-672.

Howard, B. (2014). Doctors with four Legs. *Alternative medicine: Your guide to stress relief, healing, nutrition, and more.* New York, NY: Time Books.

Holzel, B.K., Carmody, J., Vangel, M., Congleton, C., Yerramsetti, S.M., Gard, T., & Lazar, S.W. (2011). Mindfulness practice leads to increase in regional gray matter density. *Psychiatry Resources,* 191 (1), 36-43.

Hutchinson, M.G. (1985). *Transforming body-image: Learning to love the body you have.* Freedom, Ca: The Crossing Press.

Hyman, M. (2012). *The blood sugar solution: The ultrahealthy program for losing weight, preventing disease, and feeling great now!* New York, NY: Little, Brown, and Company.

Iazetto, D. (1989). *When the body is not an easy place to be: Women's sexual abuse and eating problems.* Doctoral dissertation, UECU; Yellow Springs, Ohio.

Inhelder, B. & Piaget, J. (1958). *The growth of logical thinking from childhood to adolescence.* New York, NY: Basic Books, Inc.

Institute for Natural Resources. (1994). Seminar - *Mind, mood, and appetite.* Sioux Falls, SD.

Institute for Natural Resources. (2012). Seminar - *Food Addictions, overeating, and mood swings.* Sioux Falls, SD.

Jacobson, E. (1938). *Progressive relaxation.* Chicago: University of Chicago Press.

Kabot-Zinn, J. (1990). *Full catastrophe living: Using the wisdom of your body and mind to face stress, pain, and illness.* New York, NY: Delacorte Press.

Kaplan, J.A. (1980). *A woman's conflict: The special relationship between women and food.* Englewood Cliffs, NJ: Prentice Hall Inc.

Kearney-Cooke, A. (1988). Group treatment of sexual abuse among women with eating disorders. *Women and Therapy,* 7, 5-21.

Keltner, J. (2013). *Project Awe.* John Templeton Foundation.

Kilbourne, J. (1979). *Still killing us softly.* Cambridge, MA: Cambridge Documentary Films Inc.

Kroll, S. (2017). *Acceptance and commitment therapy for substance abuse, eating disorders, anxiety, depression, self-injury, PTSD, psychosis, and more.* Workshop, Vyne Education, Sioux Falls, SD.

Levine, M.P. (1985). *The role of culture in the cause of eating disorders.* Kenyon College Alumni Bulliton, 9, 8-13.

Liu, R.T. (2017). The microbiome as a novel paradigm in studying stress and mental health. *American Psychologist,* 72 (7), 655-667.

Ludwig, D. (2016). *Always hungry: Conquer cravings, retrain your fat cells, and lose weight permanently.* New York, NY: Grand Central Life & Style.

Maine, M. (2004). *Fathers, daughters, and the pursuit of thinness.* Gurze books: Carlsbad, CA.

Marlatt, G.A. & Gordon, J.R. (EDs.), (1985). *Relapse prevention.* New York, NY: Guilford Press.

McBee, L. (2016). *Mindfulness-based stress reduction.* Workshop presented by PESI, Sioux Falls, SD.

McKay, M. & Fanning, P. (1987). *Self-esteem: A proven program of cognitive techniques for assessing, improving, and maintaining your self-esteem.* Oakland, CA: New harbinger Publications.

McManus, V. (2004). *A look in the mirror: Freeing yourself from the body-image blues.* Washington, DC: Child & Family Press.

McGraw, P. (2003). *The ultimate weight solution: The 7 keys to weight loss freedom.* New York, NY: Free Press.

Meichenbaum, D. (1985). *Stress inoculation training.* New York, NY: Pergamon Press.

Meiselman, K. (1990). *Resolving the trauma of incest: Reintegration therapy with survivors.* San Francisco: Jossey-bass.

Naimen, R. (2015). *The Sleep Secret.* Lecture [online], Institute of Integrative Nutrition, New York.

Neff, K. (2011). *Self-compassion: Stop beating yourself up and leave security behind.* Britain: Hodder and Stroughten.

O'brien, J.D. (1987). The effects of incest on female adolescent development. *Journal of the American Academy of Psychoanalysis,* 15, 88-32.

Orbach, S. (1979). *Fat is a feminist issue.* Feltham: Hamlyn Publishing.

Orbach, S. (1982). *Fat is a feminist issue TT.* New York, NY: Berkley Books.

Orbach, S. (1986). *Hunger strike: The anorexic's struggle as a metaphor for our age.* New York, NY: W.W. Norton.

Park, A. (2014). Your friendly microbes. *Alternative Medicine: Your guide to stress relief, healing, nutrition, and more.* New York, NY: Time Books.

Perlmutter, D. (2013). *Grain brain: The surprising truth about wheat, carbs, and sugar – your brain's silent killers.* New York, NY: Little, Brown and Company.

Pershing, A. (2014). *Understanding binge-eating disorder.* Lecture [online], Institute of Integrative Nutrition, New York.

Rauste von Wright, M. (1988). Body image satisfaction in adolescent girls and boys: A longitudinal study. *Journal of Youth and Adolescence,* 18 (1), 71-83.

Richards, P.S., Hardman, R.K., & Berrett, M.E. (2007). *Spiritual approaches in the treatment of women with eating disorders.* Washington DC: American Psychological Association.

Rodin, J. & Striegel-Moore, R.H. (1984). *Predicting attitudes toward body weight and food intake in women.* Paper presented at the 14th congress of the European Association of Behavior Therapy.

Romeo, F. (1984). Adolescence, sexual conflict, and anorexia nervosa. *Adolescence,* 19 (75), 551-555.

Root, M. (1987). An eight-week group treatment program for bulimia. *Journal of College Student Psychotherapy,* 4, 105-119.

Root, M. (1989). Treatment failures: The role of sexual victimization in women's addictive behaviors. *American Orthopsychiatric Association,* 4, 542-549.

Root, M. & Fallon, P. (1988). The incidence of victimization experiences in a bulimic sample. *Journal of Interpersonal Violence,* 3, 161-173.

Root, M., Fallon, P., & Friedrich, W.N. (1986). *Bulimia: A systems approach to treatment.* New York, NY: W.W. Norton.

Rosenthol, J. (2014). *Integrative nutrition: Feed your hunger for health and happiness.* New York, NY: Institute for Integrative Nutrition.

Rosenthol, J. (2015). *Integrative nutrition health coaching.* Lecture [online], Institute of Integrative Nutrition.

Roth, G. (1983). *Feeding the hungry heart.* New York, NY: New American Library.

Sark. (1992). *Inspirational Sandwich: Stories to inspire your creative freedom.* Celestial Arts: Berkeley, CA.

Schmidt, K., Cowen, P.J., Tzortziz, G., Errington, S., & Burnet, P.W.J. (2015). Prebiotic intake reduces the waking cortisol response and alters emotional bias in healthy volunteers. *Psychopharmacology, 232,* 1793-1801. http//dx.doi.org/10.1007/s00213-014-3810-0

Schwartz, M. & Gay, P. (1996). Physical and sexual abuse and neglect and eating disorder symptoms. In M.F. Schwartz and L.Cohen (Eds.) *Sexual abuse and eating disorders* (pp. 92-108). New York, NY: Brunner/Mazel.

Scully, D., Kremer, J., Meade, M.M., Graham, R., Dudgeon, K. (2011). Physical exercise and psychological well being: A critical review. *British Journal of Sports Medicine, 32* (2), 111-120.

Shroyer-Small, L. (1992). *Eating disorders and negative sexual experiences: The effectiveness of a multidimensional treatment approach on treatment outcome.* Doctoral dissertation. University of South Dakota.

Siegel, B. (2014). *Master the art of Living.* Lecture [online], Institute of Integrative Nutrition, New York.

Siegel, D. (2017). Neuroscience and therapy: The craft of rewiring the brain. *Psychotherapy Networker* (1), 45, 68.

Slade, P.D., Dewey, M.E., Newton, T., Browdie, D., Kiemle, G. (1989). Development of and preliminary validation of the body satisfaction scale. *Journal of Psychology and Health,* 4(3), 213-220.

Small, L. & Jackson, P. (1989). *Negative sexual experiences in a clinical sample of eating disordered patients.* Unpublished raw data.

Sokul, A., Goldbacher, E., McClure, K., and McMahon, C. Interoceptive awareness and emotional eating: The role of appetite and emotional awareness. *Society of Behavioral Medicine.* LaSalle University, Philadelphia, PA. https://www.sbm.org/userfiles/file/papersession4- Sokul.pdf

Sperly, M. (1987). *"The image and uses of the body in psychic conflict."* Paper presented at the Psychoanalysis Association of New York, June, 1987.

Stellar, J. (2015). Feeling awe may be good for your health. *Scientific American, 9.*

Stone, R. (2013). *Eat with joy: Redeeming God's gift of food.* Downers Grove, IL: InterVarsity Press.

Sternberg, B. (2010). *Women's health and physical fitness.* Institute for Natural Resources, homestudy.

Taitz, J. (2012). *End emotional eating: Using dialectical behavior therapy skills to cope with difficult emotions and develop a healthy relationship with food.* Oakland CA: New Harbinger Publications.

Talbott, L., Maguen, S., Epel, E.S., Metzler, T.J., & Neylan, T.C. (2013). Posttraumatic stress is associated with emotional eating. *Journal of Traumatic Stress, 26* (4), 521-525.

Thompson, J.K. (1990). *Body image disturbance – assessment and treatment.* New York, NY: Pergamon Press.

Thompson, J.K. & Psaltis, K. (1988). Multiple aspects and correlates of body figure ratings: A replication and extension of Fallon and Rozin (1985). *International Journal of Eating Disorders, 7,* 813-818.

Torem, M. (1987). Ego state therapy for eating disorders. *American Journal of Clinical Hypnosis, 30,* 94-103.

Tribole, E. & Resch, E. (2012). *Intuitive eating: A revolutionary program that works.* New York, NY: St. Martin's Griffin.

Turner, L. (1990). Weight Maintenance and Relapse Prevention. *Nutrition Clinics, 5* (1).

Van der kolk, B. (2014). *The body keeps the score: Brain, mind, and body in the healing of trauma.* New York, NY: Penguin Books.

Van der kolk, B., McFarlane, A.C., & Weisaeth, L. (1995). *Traumatic stress: The effects of overwhelming experience on mind, body, and society.* New York, NY: Guilford Publications.

Volkow, N.D., Wang, G.J., Fowler, J.S., Telang, F. (2008). Overlapping neuronal circuits in addiction and obesity: evidence of systems pathology. Philosophical Transactions R Soc London B Sci. Oct 12; 363(1507):3191-3200.

Wang, G.J., Volkow, N.D., Thanos, P.K., & Fowler, J.S. (2009). Imaging of brain dopamine pathways: Implications for understanding obesity. *Journal of Addiction Medicine,* 3 (1), 8-11.

Warren, R., Amen, D., & Hyman, M. (2013). *The Daniel plan: 40 days to a healthier life.* Grand Rapids, Michigan: Zondervan.

Watkins, J.G. (1978). Ego state therapy. In J.G. Watkins (Eds.). *The therapeutic self,* (pp.360-398). New York, NY: Science Press.

Weaver, L. (2015). *Elimination and Detoxification.* Lecture [online], Institute of Integrative Nutrition, New York.

Williams, D. (2011). *Wheat belly: Lose the wheat, lose the weight, and find your path back to health.* New York, NY: Rodale.

Woititz, J. (1983). *Adult children of alcoholics.* Florida: Health Communications.

Waterhouse, D. (1993). *Outsmarting the female fat cell: The first weight-control program designed specifically for women.* New York, NY: Hyperion.

Waterhouse, D. (1998). *Outsmarting the midlife fat cell: Winning weight control strategies for women over 35 to stay fit through menopause.* New York, NY: Hyperion.

Witkiewitz, K. & Malrlatt, G.A. (2004). Relapse prevention for alcohol and drug problems. *American Psychologist,* 59 (4), 224-235.

Wooley, S. & Kearney-Cooke, A. (1986). Intensive treatment of bulimia and body-image disturbances. In K. Brownell and J. Foreyt (EDs.) *Handbook of eating disorders,* (pp. 477-502). New York: Basic Books, Inc.

Wooley, S.C. & Lewis, K. G. (1989). The missing woman: Intensive family oriented treatment of bulimia. *Journal of Feminist Family Therapy,* 1, 61-83.

Wooley, S. C. & Wooley, O.W. (1986). Thinness mania. *American Health,* 10, 68-74.